DEADLY PYRE

A Kelly McKay Medical Thriller
Book One — Seattle
by
Betty Kuffel

Table of Contents

DEADLY PYRE

This book is a work of fiction. References to real locations, real people, names, characters or places are used fictitiously. Resemblances to actual events, places or persons, living or dead, are coincidental.

Published in the U.S.A.

Montana Sunrise Books Publisher

Copyright © 2018 by Montana Sunrise Books

Author: Betty Kuffel

All rights reserved.

No part of this book may be used or reproduced in any manner without written permission of the author, except in brief quotations within reviews.

For information contact montanasunrisebooks@gmail.com

Website: http://www.bettykuffel.com

DEDICATION
For Jenna
An aspiring author

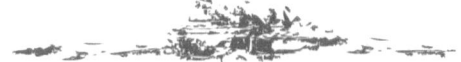
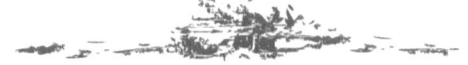

DEADLY PYRE

Chapter 1 Trauma Code

The approaching siren ricocheted off tall buildings. Red ambulance lights pulsed the nocturnal Seattle fog outside Harbor ER where the charge nurse and I waited, ready for the challenge of an unconscious young addict with a chest stab wound. Trauma codes occurred several times a day at the University of Washington teaching hospital. Outside in cool air for a few minutes relieved my exhaustion. Only seven hours to go before sleep, and six months to go before the end of ER medical training.

Ambulance back doors flung open in a cloud of diesel exhaust before the vehicle came to a stop. A young paramedic pumped on the stabbing victim's chest with one hand and moved the stretcher toward us. "Dr. McKay, the stab wound is in the left chest. First Responders started CPR."

His partner clamped the mask tighter and squeezed a bag pushing in oxygen. "We didn't delay transport to place a tube or line. She was just around the corner on James."

Inside a large trauma bay with bright lights and equipment everywhere, I gave the gathered trauma team a rapid overview. "She's in hemorrhagic shock from a single stab wound in the left chest. Her only chance for survival is to crack her chest and stop the bleeding."

The team washed over the young victim in a wave of yellow gowns and gloved hands. We slid her to the ER bed where nurses connected monitors and readied bags of saline for IVs.

"Get her on a ventilator, two large-bore IVs, labs, high volume fluid, and pump in O negative blood." I looked around. "Where's Warren? Page him stat."

Annie's scissors chomped through ragged blue jeans. Another nurse ripped open the victim's T-shirt and peeled back her clothing.

The thin adolescent body of an intravenous drug user lay before us, mutilated by needled-tracked veins, a clitoral ring, and tarnished rings through pubescent nipples. A wad of Vaseline gauze sealed the half-inch stab wound. Blood oozed around the edge of the dressing.

An adrenalin-junkie paramedic calmly searched for an intravenous lifeline for fluids and blood. Like him, I had learned to internalize stress and remain calm under dire circumstances.

A practiced ER behavior.

Don't cry when babies die.

No emotions. Do your job.

I examined the patient while talking to staff and ran the trauma code like Jackson Hunter, our brilliant director, had drilled into me over the past two and a half years. I spoke his words. "Be careful. Protect yourselves. Anyone not assigned here, please leave."

Anesthesiology resident Dr. Milt Flora rushed into the room and elbowed his way toward the head of the bed. "Get me a goddamned tube."

I pointed at the ventilator. "You're late. We already placed the ET tube." Milt glared. His attitude made me want to tube him just to stop his insults.

Milt detested taking orders, especially from women. His surly behavior tonight reminded me of Annie's comment after one of his fits during a prior code. She said, "What do you expect, Kelly? His father is a cop and his mother a psychiatrist. The poor guy was probably potty-trained at gunpoint."

Annie, a striking black woman who had worked at Harbor for years, took charge of nursing issues. The medics helped us stabilize patients by adding another layer of expertise to our rapid ER interventions until they had to rush off on another call. Paramedic Nate grabbed a gown and gloves. "What do you want me to do Doc?"

"Start a peripheral line if you can find a vein while I place a large-bore line in her internal jugular."

His fingers searched the patient's arms for an intravenous site. "She's hard-core. Needle tracks everywhere. Her veins feel like ropes." His initial grim expression flashed to a smile. "She'd have trouble using this one." He scrubbed the skin over a pristine vein on her upper arm with an alcohol wipe and eased in an intracath needle and short plastic tube. Blood flashed back.

RNs connected blood and saline via rapid infusers into the medic's line and the line I placed in the victim's neck. "Pump in six units of blood and get six more of O negative while we're waiting for type-specific units."

Annie opened a surgical tray and placed it on a stand next to me on the patient's left side.

Milt smirked from the head of the table. He monitored the patient's airway, oxygen status and fluids. "What are you, McKay, a one-man show? Where's your surgeon?"

My redhead temper flared. I clenched my teeth to stop words I might regret. I would have preferred doing a vasectomy on Milt without anesthetic, but the asshole did have a point. "Where the hell is Dr. Warren? Page him again!"

I would have to answer to Dr. Hunter if I didn't follow protocol and opened the teenager's chest without a surgeon to assist. But, the patient would lose her chance for survival if I didn't act quickly. I'd have hell to pay either way. "Stop chest compressions. Check vital signs."

Milt announced, "We made a little progress. Weak carotid pulse. Heart rate 130. She's had five units of packed red cells and four liters of saline."

My gut hurt and hands shook as I pulled on sterile gloves. "Okay. Let's open."

Annie removed the Vaseline gauze and scrubbed the victim's chest with iodine solution. Each ventilator breath spewed red droplets from the stab wound. The blood mixed with the smelly brown liquid, forming glistening copper streaks in an abstract mosaic on the white and purple mottled skin.

Annie handed a male med student sterile gloves. "You're Dr. McKay's assistant."

His eyes glistened as if she had given a kid a bag of chocolates.

We draped and clipped sterile sheets over the patient, covering all but the left chest.

I gave my assistant the suction and poised the scalpel at the point of incision. "Get ready. We'll have torrential bleeding when I open."

Milt's eyes squinted at me above his mask. "I have two units up and two more ready to hang. You should wait for help."

"There's no time. Somebody page a surgeon, anyone!"

One swift strike along the rib interspace below the stab wound, beneath the breast, extending from sternum to underarm, opened her chest. A geyser of blood shot over my unprotected arms and sloshed my blue scrub top.

I had warned everyone else, but I had failed to wear a protective gown myself—a critical oversight in my rush to help an addict likely to carry a blood-borne dreaded disease. I couldn't take the time to put on a gown with her chest open.

The clear plastic suction hose turned crimson and filled a canister.

Milt scrambled to hang more blood.

I slid rib spreaders into the incision and spun the crank to separate the blades, opening the chest wide. The student suctioned more blood.

Someone pushed in beside me.

I couldn't look away from what I was doing to see who it was, but I hoped it was Brett Warren. When I heard the voice, I cringed.

Mona Maddox, another senior ER resident, peered into the chest. Her harsh personality always raised my blood pressure. "Kelly, I'll help you. What's the history?" She dived into a gown and gloves.

I gave her a mini history while I suctioned, trying to clear the blood inside the chest to expose the bleeding site while Mona's shrill voice twisted the emotions of those near her, much like Milt's voice did. Having both of them on this team added to the chaos. Her first demand to Annie was, "Scalpel!"

Annie cautiously passed a scalpel to her.

Mona elbowed me. "I'm going to extend the incision a little to give us more visibility."

I adjusted the rib spreader and felt a sudden sharp pain. I jerked back my hand.

A slice through my glove across the back of my hand ran red. I felt blood pooling inside my glove. "Dammit, Mona, you cut me. This is an addict!"

Blood dripped off my gloved fingertips to the floor.

Mona snarled, "I told you I was extending the wound. It's your fault for getting in the way."

She pushed me with her ample hip. "Get a new glove and give me some damn help."

The horror of my cut awash with an addict's blood sent fear to my core. A major blood contamination from an addict. HIV? Hepatitis C? I flexed my fingers to be sure the tendons were intact and could still grip an instrument.

The worried eyes of the team watched an RN remove my bloody glove and slosh iodine over the laceration. They understood that prolonged contact between the addict's blood and my open wound increased the risk of blood-borne disease.

Annie held open a fresh sterile glove. I plunged in my hand. She offered a second as a double barrier.

Milt screamed, "We're losing ground! Her pressure's 60! Set up the reinfuser! More blood, stat!" A nurse moved to the head of the table to help him pump fluids into the patient, and she hung another unit of packed red blood cells.

Mona grabbed a suction from the med student's hand and pulled off the angled metal handle to provide a larger opening for removing the blood. She thrust the tube deep in the chest.

Profuse bleeding made it impossible to see the cut vessel. I scooped out blood with my hands, soaking my shirt and pant legs. Warm liquid and clots slithered off the gurney onto the floor, squishing inside my shoes.

"We can't see!" Mona yelled. "Somebody adjust the damn light."

A bright beam swung around and aimed directly into the red cavern. I pushed a soft gray lung out of the way and felt the staccato hammering of the patient's heart. In the depths of the chest, a small area of rhythmic bursts burbled up like water from an artesian well. I blindly squeezed the submerged vessel with my left hand.

Mona pushed against me. "Let me see." She pressed on my lacerated hand.

I gasped with pain. "Mona, move your head. You're in my way." I held out my injured hand to Annie. "Vascular clamp!"

A clamp slapped my hand. "Mona, suction by my left hand so I can see what I'm clamping."

She suctioned but blocked my view again. I nudged her with my hip. "I can't get a clamp around the vessel if I can't see it. Give me some room."

Mona held out her hand. "I see a gusher. Clamp! Give me a clamp!"

An operating room tech who had just arrived to help passed Mona a long vascular clamp.

I held firm, compressing the bleeding vessel.

Mona struggled inside the chest, suctioning. She clicked the clamp closed.

I loosened my hold.

Blood spurted. She had missed.

I squeezed again, stopping the flow. I would have done better without her. I held out my hand for another long vascular clamp.

Milt barked orders to two nurses helping him pump in blood.

Still controlling a bleeding site with my left hand, Mona took the suction to clear the area.

I clamped. The bleeding stopped. I took a deep breath and let go.

No spurting.

The bleeding stopped, but not because I'd clamped the vessel. Her heart quivered against my hand.

No rhythmic contractions.

I squeezed an empty heart. We'd lost. "Stop resuscitation. She bled out." My eyes went to the wall clock. "Time of death, zero-zero-thirty."

A blood-soaked pant leg clung to my skin like a hand.

The phantom grip of the dead girl.

In my mind, her voice cried out, "Doc, don't stop. Help me."

I stepped away from the bed. My foot slipped on the bloody floor, sending me off balance. I grabbed Mona's arm to keep from falling. Perspiration moistened my forehead. Rivulets of sweat joined the red stains soaking my scrub shirt.

The wordless trauma team removed gloves and long-sleeved gowns in slow motion as they backed away from the grisly scene. Eyes drifted to my scrub top stuck to my skin like in a wet T-shirt contest. Milt met my eyes then fixated on my breasts.

The cardiac monitor displayed the undulating, useless electrical rhythm of the teenager's fibrillating heart.

Milt turned off the ventilator and IV pumps.

The monitor screen went dark.

The oxygen flow stopped.

My voice sounded loud in the silent room. "Thanks for your help. We didn't get to her in time."

Milt's final statement before the door closed behind him, "What we needed was a *real* surgeon."

The rest of the staff filed out, leaving me with Mona, Annie, and the body.

Mona disconnected bloody suction tubing from a canister. She stared at the dead girl while slowly coiling the tube like a lasso.

Her presence was worse than no help. I tried to sound grateful, hiding the anger I felt. "Thanks for the help."

"You really blew it, getting that laceration, Kelly. I'll stitch it for you." Mona threw the coil into a metal bucket with a loud clang like an exclamation point at the end of her statement. "Milt's an ass. Besides, I knew we couldn't save her. I wouldn't have tried if I'd been in charge." She removed her gloves and gown. "Get your baseline labs drawn and start HIV prophylaxis tonight. That loser's blood could kill you."

"I haven't forgotten and won't forget you did this to me." I walked to the sink and removed my gloves to clean the wound. "I'll have someone else stitch it."

Mona scowled and walked out.

Chapter 2 Exposure

Exposed white extensor tendons lay like fat spaghetti within the three-inch cut across the back of my hand. The cut didn't worry me. A nick in one of the tendons required no repair, but the blood exposure mandated immediate drugs. Contaminated needle sticks are low risk for disease transmission, but a large wound with blood contact upped my chances of developing a fatal disease.

My life as an ER doctor would be over if I contracted HIV or hepatitis C. I didn't want to think about it.

The cold water ran red. I scrubbed the wound with a surgical prep sponge. It hurt like hell until I injected anesthetic to dull the pain.

Annie irrigated the bleeding wound with two liters of sterile saline and compressed a wad of gauze over the surface with an elastic wrap. "Do you want me to order a stat HIV and hepatitis panel on the patient's blood?"

"Yes and have them come down a little later and draw a baseline on my blood. I hope they have some of the patient's blood from the first draw. We gave her so many units, we'd get a dilutional false negative from a later draw even if she was positive for disease." I slumped on a stool near the ER bed and put on clean gloves for a post-mortem exam. "Taking care of critical patients when I'm this tired is insane."

"It went well except for Mona. I can't believe she slashed you in her stupidity. What was she doing here tonight?"

"I think she's still on a cardiology elective. Must miss the ER." I looked at the gaping chest incision. "I would have done better without her but I'm not sure we could have saved this patient even with Warren helping."

From the opposite side of the bed, Annie looked at the victim's face. "She was here a couple weeks ago. Medics found her lethargic in a flophouse on Broadway. Beat up. One eye swollen shut. You can still see some discoloration on her face, here." Annie pointed.

"Do you remember what her drug screen showed?"

"Positive for benzos, narcotics, and meth. The two friends with her that night looked just like her. Hair dyed black. Heads partially shaved. Facial piercings and many earrings."

"Probably had piercings in other body parts like hers."

Annie nodded. "Those kids look so much alike, it's hard to tell boys from girls until you look between their legs."

I pointed out the vascular anatomy and injury to Annie. "The stab got both the pulmonary artery and the aorta. I guess Mona was right. Based on these injuries, there is no way we could have saved her."

"You didn't know that when you had to make the decision to open her. I've only seen a couple of patients saved by an ER thoracotomy in the fifteen years I've worked here." Annie turned the flaccid body so I could re-examine the victim's back. "It would have been nice to have the surgical resident here, but you couldn't wait. This went fast, like it's supposed to." After my exam, Annie turned the body back and purified the death scene with a white sheet.

"I wonder why Brett didn't show up."

"Brett's not the most reliable doc around here. He's missed codes before and can be a hothead."

"I hope he's cool this morning when Hunter burns him in critique for not showing up."

The disgusting red stains on my pale blue scrubs were drying at the edges. I pulled the sticky part of a pant leg away from my skin and again felt the clinging sensation on my leg. "These scrubs feel gross. I have to shower and find someone to stitch my hand before the anesthetic wears off."

"I'll see if Lynn Cabot can do it for you. I'm glad you refused Mona's offer." Annie handed me a gown. "Put this on to cover yourself. You can't walk through the ER looking like you work in a slaughterhouse."

I tied the gown around me. "Somebody out there didn't like this unfortunate girl."

Annie poured hydrogen peroxide over our shoes to clean off some of the blood. "Broadway used to be a nice district with great restaurants, but I wouldn't go there at night after what we've seen recently. This is the second addict homicide I've seen in the past two weeks."

Blood dripped off the bed onto the floor in a gelatinous dinner plate-sized clot. Red footprints tracked the room. Towels, instruments, suction canisters, all red.

Annie handed me a pair of shoe covers to avoid tracking blood into the hallway. "We have to remember to put these on *before* we meet the ambulances." She pulled the privacy curtain across the doorway to block the view into the room.

The door clicked shut behind us.

A nurse met us in the hallway. "Dr. McKay, the police are here to talk to you about this patient."

Annie shook her head. "She has to get cleaned up. I'll talk to them while she showers. Do we have an open suture bay?"

The nurse raised her eyebrows, eyes focusing on my bandaged hand.

Annie explained about the laceration.

"I'm so sorry, Dr. Mc Kay. I'll set one up. A med student could suture it for you. Is that okay?"

"Sure. It'll take me a few minutes to shower." I walked down the hall, my feet squishing with each step.

Seattle Police Detective Cy Jones caught up to me as I tried to escape. His usual twinkling eyes turned dark when he saw the legs of my scrubs below the gown. "I can see why you're rushing off."

"I'm anxious to shower and get this drug-user's blood washed off."

"What's wrong with your hand?"

"Scalpel cut contaminated with her blood."

"That's horrible. What if she had HIV?"

"We have good drugs and I'll start them tonight, but I'm worried. After I shower, we can talk about the victim. It'll take a few extra minutes to get some stitches."

"I'll have a cup of coffee ready. You look like you need one."

"I do. Annie said she'd go into the room with you now if you want to get started."

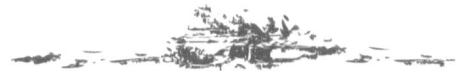

Mona sat in the locker room sipping coffee and reading *People* magazine.

I stripped off clothing as soon as I entered. "I was surprised to see you here tonight. Aren't you on an elective?"

"It's my last night on cardiology. I have to come back to this stinking place in the morning." Mona tossed her magazine onto a table. "I'm leaving now to get some sleep. I came in to use the library when I heard the stat page for Brett."

"I wonder where he is."

Mona watched me remove my bloody shoes and toss them in the trash. "I saw him in the library. Maybe he fell asleep."

I looked down at the red stains on my skin. "It's been a long, ugly day."

"It'll be better when we start working twelves on January first instead of twenty-four-hour shifts." The door closed behind her.

I threw my underwear in the garbage.

Warm swirls of antibacterial soap mixed with red-tinged water rushed down the drain. My legs and feet returned to pale freckled skin. I shampooed my hair. My tense muscles relaxed. I wanted to stay in the shower for an hour.

The numb area and bandage on my hand reminded me of the possible consequences I faced. I removed the glove I'd used to protect the wound from the shower and donned fresh scrubs. Scratchy seams against my bare skin increased my desire to be home in bed wearing soft PJs, but I had hours more to work. I rushed back, dreading the thought of discussing my dire situation with Dr. Jackson after morning report and, even worse, of having to fight off some incurable disease.

The med student added more anesthetic, irrigated my wound, and closed the edges in record time. In the dictation room, Cy looked up with his characteristic smile that had brightened some of my darkest ER shifts. "Hey, Kelly, that was a fast shower and change. I like that curly wet hairdo." He handed me coffee. "I'll microwave it if it's too cold."

"Thanks. It's okay. I've learned to like it cold."

"The medical examiner will be happy to see you didn't cut through the stab wound. It'll help him identify the type of blade."

"I know that's standard procedure in possible homicides. Are you finished with your investigation here?"

"Yeah. You can send the body to the morgue for the medical examiner. The ME will want all tubes left in place since it's a homicide. We also bagged her hands to preserve potential evidence. Did you see any defensive wounds?"

"None. Only the stab wound, needle-tracked arms, and an old facial bruise."

Cy took a few notes. "Did the medics say if she talked to them?"

"She was unresponsive. Never regained consciousness. Cracking her chest was her only chance, but we couldn't save her."

"You can't save 'em all, Kelly."

"I know, but we try. Her stab wound hit two major vessels."

He eyed my bandaged hand. "I'm worried about your cut."

"Me, too. I hope she's clean."

Annie entered the room carrying a packet of pills. "Kelly, take these, the sooner the better." She thrust them at me. "We keep one dose on hand in the ER for major blood exposures. I think you're the first one in months."

I accepted the pills and swallowed them with lukewarm coffee. "That's an ignominious honor. Thanks."

"This is the second druggie death from a chest wound I've seen in ER in the past couple weeks." Annie addressed Detective Jones, "Aren't you investigating the other one, too?"

"Yes, and there's a third. All are female teens from the Broadway District."

Annie's parting words were, "Good luck finding the guy."

I swished and swallowed the dregs of my coffee to rid my mouth of the pill taste. Cy listened while I dictated. He took a few notes. I ended the dictation after a spiel of medical information, description of physical findings, and interventions.

Cy sat back in his chair. "You do talk fast. I don't even think that fast."

"If I didn't, I'd spend even more time in this damned cubicle."

The detective checked his notes. "What injuries did you find from the stab?"

"The knife penetrated both the pulmonary artery and the aorta."

"The ME called me a few days ago. Injuries in the first two homicides were similar. If this makes three, we may have a serial killer."

Cy's comment left me chilled. "Who would do this to an unfortunate group of young women?"

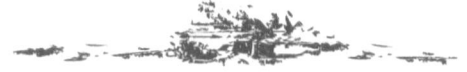

"Trauma code, ER. Trauma code, ER." An overhead page sounded, and my beeper fired off. Seconds later, other ER staff pagers sounded. We met at the desk for a radio report from the flight team. A male RN arriving with me said, "I love working with you, Dr. McKay. You're a disaster magnet. We haven't had time to clean up the mess from the last one and here we are again."

"Are you ready?"

He smiled. "Love it. I'm always ready for more."

Staff members stood around the desk listening to the flight nurse's disconcerting radio report. He requested a hot unload for an unconscious young woman with airway problems. She had sustained facial, head, and chest trauma in a T-bone car accident.

A survey of the trauma team concerned me, too. "The chopper's only two minutes out. General surgery and anesthesia aren't here yet. Page them again."

Annie suggested, "Should we alert the OR and ask for neurosurgery to respond?"

I agreed and walked toward the ambulance entrance. The doors gaped, as if sensing my need to disappear into the night and find a warm place to sleep, a different job, a different life. A life where I didn't face the daily threat of exposure to deadly disease and violence.

I couldn't help wondering if the choice of a different job might already be out of my hands because of the contaminated wound.

This time, I wore a long-sleeved protective gown, gloves, and shoe covers. The black sky pelted my face with light rain. A wind swirled coastal fog inland, clearing the lights of downtown and sending a chill through my damp hair.

Harbor Medical Center and many other healthcare facilities perched along Seattle's First Hill had straight routes down Skid Road. Instead of skidding logs as in the early days of the city, many down-and-out homeless people lived in the Skid Road area of Pioneer Square. Noise from the freeway traffic below rose to greet me. A distant siren cut through the din, nearing James Street. A turn up the steep grade could carry them to us. In moments, its urgent tone diminished as it passed by and was absorbed by the night.

Droplets clung to my face like cold beads of sweat. Cigarette smoke rising above a security guard standing out of the rain near the hospital entrance polluted my air. Inside, the trauma team dressed in flowing yellow gowns milled silently near the door, mouths opening and closing in soundless conversation like goldfish in a bowl.

Standing outside for a few minutes allowed me to experience the elements while waiting for the case to arrive. The cold air cleared my brain and beat back the exhaustion from being trapped inside with ailing humanity for so many hours. A short break provided a few moments to reflect on the reported injuries and anticipate rapid interventions we might need to perform on the arriving patient.

Northward across the parking lot, three staff members tensed against the wind and huddled beneath an overhang near the helipad. The pulsing rotor noise materialized from the west, and I watched them twist their heads in unison toward the sound like robots. Our eyes searched the dark sky for flashing lights.

Wind generated by the noisy chopper blasted the waiting workers as the helicopter settled onto the tarmac. The engine noise abated. The older-model Augusta helicopter had no rotor brake, and the patient was too unstable to wait for the blades to stop turning before unloading. The flight crew had asked for a hot unload, so the staff advanced, heads down, as the large blades spun overhead. Fumes carried by rotor wash swept toward me.

The skilled pilot had braved the bad weather, helping the medical team use their battlefield experience to save lives. The flight nurse popped the side door of the helicopter open and peered out. He shielded his face from wet air stirred by the blades and jumped to the ground. The two flight personnel pulled their loaded stretcher onto a wheeled gurney supplied by the ground team. Staff surrounded the patient and wheeled her at a fast jog toward the ER entrance. I advanced to help them and hear their report.

Blood- and rain-soaked jumpsuits plastered the bodies of the disheveled former army nurse and ex-LA paramedic. The flight nurse wiped his forehead on a sleeve. "Hi, Dr. McKay. She is critical and the cuff on her ET tube has a leak."

His paramedic partner held the tube securely and squeezed the bag as we ran. "It was a difficult intubation. She has facial fractures and had a lot of blood in her airway, so we didn't want to attempt a new tube and chance losing the airway."

The ER doors parted for the entourage. The trauma team swept forward to help. A gown draped Brett Warren's tall frame. "Hi, Brett, I guess this one is yours."

His handsome face tensed. "I guess it is, Kelly. I owe you big time after the last case. Sorry I missed the page."

I acknowledged his apology, and we turned our attention to the unconscious woman, her face bruised, eyes swollen shut, long brown hair matted with blood. Frothy red fluid sprayed from her mouth with each squeeze of the oxygen bag. She needed a better airway, and fast.

Interventions similar to the last trauma code proceeded. The flight nurse handed airway management over to Milt Flora. In one quick move, Milt jerked out the poorly functioning tube and the woman's blood-spattering respirations stopped.

I took a deep breath and held it, a method I used to help me time a patient without oxygen. If I had to take a breath, she should, too. I looked at the wall clock and watched Milt's attempts to clear her bloody airway and replace the tube. He swept a broken tooth from her mouth and suctioned again.

She had no respiratory effort.

Seconds passed.

I had to take another breath.

I watched the heart monitor. Brett said, "Milt, her heart rate is fifty. Get the tube in or she'll have a cardiac arrest."

A student at my side asked, "Why the slow heart rate? Shouldn't it be racing?"

"You're right." I watched the sweep of the second hand as I explained. "A slow heart rate is a bad sign under these circumstances. The heart may slow for many reasons, but two common causes are severe brain injury and a heart failing from lack of oxygen. In her case, maybe both."

"Milt, two minutes without oxygen." To the student, I said, "Once he gets the tube in, we'll see if her heart rate picks up."

Brett and I quickly assessed her injuries.

Milt wedged her mouth open with the scope and suctioned her throat to help visualize her vocal cords for proper tube placement. The flight nurse stabilized the patient's head to decrease movement and avoid further injury if she had a neck fracture. Milt suctioned again. "I can't see a thing. There's too much blood." His frustration showed as he slammed the scope onto the bed by the patient's head.

I looked at the clock and took another breath. "Three minutes; three minutes without an airway." Dr. Hunter's unmerciful tirades over delayed airway placements disturbed my focus. There'd be hell to pay.

Sweat ran down Milt's face. He shook his head. Pulled out his misplaced tube and tried again. Brett and I palpated her chest for injury. Checked her heart and belly. Milt prepared for another try.

Brett put on sterile gloves. "This is way too long, Milt. I'm doing a surgical airway."

The ex-military flight nurse edged closer to Milt. "This was a tough intubation for us in the field. Mind if I give it a try?"

I hoped Milt would accept help from the skilled flight nurse, though in Milt's eyes, nurses were subordinates.

Airway is first priority. All other interventions are for naught if there's no oxygen to the brain.

Milt listened to him—after all, it was another male who was offering help. "I'll give you some cric pressure. Brett, if we don't get it in this time, go ahead and cut."

Annie opened the surgical kit and swabbed the patient's neck. Brett stood ready with scalpel in hand.

Milt pushed down on the patient's neck to move the trachea into better view to help the RN for this one last try.

Sometimes, in dire situations, teaching opportunities were buried in chaos and the medical students learned from participating or just watching. With Brett in charge of this patient, I had time to give explanations to the two medical students assigned to the team. "Because of unstable face fractures and bleeding into her airway, an oxygen mask is ineffective. The surgical procedure Dr. Warren will use cuts through the cricothyroid membrane, a *cric* for short. That's the quickest and least bloody way to enter the trachea and directly place a tube for oxygen delivery."

Brett watched Milt and the flight nurse struggle. X-ray techs readied film cassettes and waited for a cue from Dr. Warren. He called, "Type and cross six units. Get a blood gas. Chest and pelvis X-rays. Everybody help the techs." The second Brett's blade touched the skin, the flight nurse slid a tube in.

Milt inflated the cuff around the tube and squeezed the bag. The patient's chest rose.

Success.

Brett placed the scalpel back on the tray. I listened to the woman's lungs to be sure the tube was delivering oxygen to both lung fields. "She has equal breath sounds." I explained to the students, "If it's in too far, the tube blocks one side and delivers oxygen to only one main bronchus, so you will always want to listen to both sides of a chest after tube placement."

"Congratulations on getting it in." Brett told the nurse and then turned to Milt, "You dodged the bullet, but Hunter won't like our time."

Milt glared at Brett.

The patient's heart rate increased after a couple of minutes on 100 percent oxygen.

Brett's shoulders relaxed. His facial features softened. He didn't have to cut a hole in the patient's trachea for an airway, and she was showing some improvement.

I listened to her lungs again. "Brett, her breath sounds are decreased on the left lung field. I think she has rib fractures and a pneumothorax. Do you want me to put in the chest tube?"

"Be ready to do it as soon as we get her X-rayed."

While waiting for the images, I chose my site and infiltrated anesthetic in the area between two ribs. The anesthetic was probably unnecessary because of her unresponsive state.

Holding my sterile-gloved hands away from my body, taking care not to contaminate them, I stood at Brett's side to view digital X-ray images as they appeared on the monitor. He announced, "She has a fifty percent collapse of the left lung. Like Dr. McKay said, there are at least four rib fractures with air tracking into the soft tissue." He pointed out the findings to the med students. "The X-ray shows blood and air compressing the lung. A chest tube will remove both and allow the lung to reinflate."

The students watched me cut between two ribs and push a large tube into the chest cavity. A gush of air and blood sprayed out the end before a nurse hooked it to suction. I stitched the tube in place to keep it from dislodging. With the lung re-expanding, the patient's oxygen saturation and vital signs improved, but she remained in shock after receiving four units of blood.

Brett ordered a trauma CT scan that would spiral from the head through the neck, chest, abdomen, and pelvis. It would tell us the extent of the brain and internal injuries.

I suggested the med students examine her injuries. "You can feel a soft swelling behind the left ear, then a sharp ridge. It's a definite skull fracture. Be gentle." Two students followed my instructions. "Her eyelids are swollen shut. I'll need one of you to help me open them to check her eyes and see if her pupils are reactive. Someone, please dim the lights."

Having Brett work with me on this trauma patient decreased my anxiety. I agreed with his actions, and it gave me time with the medical students. Being chief ER resident would allow me time to teach. However, after nights like this, I wondered about my sanity, applying for a job that would mean another year in the Harbor ER.

The room darkened. Brett stood with his back to us as he studied the X-rays of her pelvis. Only the soft gray light emanating from the digital viewing screen illuminated the room and outlined Brett's profile. Shadows darkened his handsome features when he turned back toward the patient.

Ophthalmoscope in hand, I leaned forward to look inside the patient's eyes. At my elbow, a student palpated her head. In the semidarkness, Brett's hands appeared to help ease open the swollen lids. We both bent forward. His face brushed mine, leaving behind a touch of sweaty scent on my skin. A warm feeling swept over me, and it wasn't the air temperature.

Pheromones in the heat of trying to save this poor woman?

Hmm. Is adrenalin a pheromone?

The woman's eyes brought me back to reality. Fish eyes. Huge pupils. Non-seeing. I directed my thoughts away from Brett and explained to the students, "Her pupils are large and unreactive, a bad sign." Fixed, dilated pupils. Dead eyes.

When the lights flipped on, it was like walking out of a matinee into bright sunlight. Brett's proximity made me feel self-conscious, as if every freckle and the hated burn scars on my neck fluoresced.

Brett sensed my discomfort and, from his smirk, enjoyed it. He looked into my eyes. A smile crossed his lips. He whispered and raised an eyebrow, "Dr. McKay, would you go with me to the CT scanner? I might need some help."

At that moment, I would have followed him almost anywhere. I hoped my expression didn't reveal my thoughts. How could I be thinking about him, when we were supposed to be focused on saving a life?

Annie and I helped move the patient to the CT suite down the hall in Radiology. With Brett in attendance, there was no necessity for me to remain, but Annie and I lingered in the dim light and studied the first few images that appeared on the monitor. Brett stood behind me, his hand resting on my shoulder. I enjoyed the proximity and envisioned another *date* with him, but not in a CT suite.

A radiologist seated at the console pointed out abnormalities as images painted the screen.

Significant bleeding in the brain.

Prospects for survival, grim.

My beeper went off. I showed Annie the number. "ER is calling us."

Brett dropped his hand from my shoulder. "I can take it from here. Thanks for the help."

On our way back to ER, Annie said, "Brett's calm, almost too nice to be a surgeon at times, but I've seen his temper."

"He did a good job tonight. I like him, but he's too good looking."

Annie glanced at me. "That's not possible."

"He's distracting."

"So I noticed."

Chapter 3 Another Victim

The packed waiting room was reduced by two after Security evicted an arguing couple. Eight gurneys occupied by drunks sat parallel parked in an alcove we called "the pit." The men exhaled alcohol fumes in a haze of dreams while awaiting transport down the street to detox. Annie commented, "It would be fun to place bets on their alcohol levels, but we're too busy tonight."

About three hours later, as I finished dictating a stack of charts, Annie stuck her head in. "Are you ready for another patient?" She placed a chart in front of me. "Our new nurse Shannon is with her."

"What's the problem?"

"A raped teenager. She might freak out with a male examiner, and Lynn Cabot is tied up with another case."

"Jamie Doe, age fourteen." I read the name and age aloud. "What's with her name?"

"She's a runaway and won't give us her last name."

Annie walked with me down the hall to a private room where a mirrored wall hid a one-way viewing window. Most ER rooms, with curtains around exam tables, provided inadequate privacy for rape exams. The hidden room with audio helped investigators during difficult assault exams.

Detectives could watch and record a physician interview without making victims undergo repeated stressful questioning.

A colorful curtain inside the door blocked the interior view from the hallway.

Annie paused outside. "I hate rape cases. They're so emotional, and we always end up in court."

"I'd go to court any time to put a rapist in prison."

Annie conceded my point and went back to work.

An attractive RN with dark hair in a loose braid dangling to her waist helped the victim. The thin teen stood on a large sheet of paper used to catch trace evidence. The nurse dropped pieces of clothing into paper bags. Purple bruises and swollen lips distorted the victim's baby face. Her hair was in a style similar to the earlier stab victim's, and her prominent dark eyes, like those of a starving feral cat, stared at me.

The nurse in designer, form-fitting scrubs finished tying the patient's gown and wrapped a warmed blanket around her shoulders before turning to me. "Hi, Dr. McKay, we haven't met. I'm Shannon. This is Jamie."

"Hello to both of you.

Jamie stared at her dirty bare feet and said nothing.

"The medics picked her up a few blocks from here after an assault. She's on the run from a bad home situation, turning tricks to feed herself."

Jamie looked through me and said nothing.

Her blank expression implied indifference, maybe intoxication. "I'm sorry this happened to you."

"I had it coming. Just do what you have to do and get me out of here."

She refused to answer most of my questions but provided some history. "A guy in a sports car picked me up by the Deluxe Tap." Jamie examined her hands. A black lace tattoo encircled her right ring finger. She gnawed on chips of purple polish clinging to dirty nails. "He flashed a fifty and I climbed in." She shrugged.

Shannon ripped open the sexual assault kit and arranged a dozen small envelopes, slides, swabs, and tubes. She labeled each item and turned on the specimen dryer. Its hum provided background noise in the otherwise silent room. She looked more like a model than an ER nurse. "You're so organized, Shannon. It looks like you've helped with a few of these."

Her voice soft, she said, "I've lost count."

Shannon motioned for Jamie to sit on the exam table. "Let's get started."

I continued asking questions. "Are you using condoms?"

"Hell, no, Doc, most guys won't use 'em." Jamie drilled me with her brown eyes. "At least I got the Depo shot so I can't get pregnant for two more months."

The hospital gown gaped open, exposing her thin buttocks. Blood smeared her crotch and dripped down her inner thighs. "I've been bleedin' more than a period." She grasped the edge of the table as she stepped up onto a stool, turned, and slowly sat down on a pad covering the end of the table. "What do you want me to do?"

"Sit while I check you over and listen to your chest. After that, you'll need to lie back." She grimaced as if expecting my next instruction. "You'll need to put your feet in the stirrups. I'll do the pelvic exam and collect fluids for the evidence kit."

Jamie jutted her jaw. "One of my friends had this done. I'm okay with everything else, but you ain't pullin' hair outta my privates." She clenched her fists. "I want that dude dead for what he did to me."

My preliminary exam revealed dirt, bruises, and bad teeth. No evidence of IV drug use or damage in her nose from cocaine. Four piercings in each ear, with some holes lacking earrings. One disfigured lobe bore a healed tear from a ripped-out earring. Skin scrapes and early bruising marked her skinny body. A life-size ladybug tattoo decorated her right ankle.

Jamie put her feet up and slid into position. "I don't shoot drugs. I've seen what they did to my mom. She's an addict."

I told her I'd be gentle and eased the warmed, lubricated speculum inside.

She yelped and jerked back in pain.

"I'm sorry we have to do this, but if he ejaculated, the vaginal tests could show DNA proof of who did this to you. I also have to look inside to see where the blood is coming from."

Jamie hid her face. "I'm sorry for being such a baby. Thanks for being nice."

Shannon handed me a UV light and darkened the room. Large smears on Jamie's pelvic area glowed fluorescent green. This visual indicated the presence of semen.

I swabbed the stains for inclusion in the rape kit collections and handed Shannon the moist swabs. "Jamie, you won't need stitches inside. Superficial tears in the mucous membrane are oozing blood, but they usually heal quickly."

Jamie remained stoic for most of the specimen collections, but her breathing was ragged.

I peered over the sheet covering her knees.

Tears welled up and spilled, forming tiny rivers trailing silty black mascara down her cheeks. She hid her face.

Shannon placed the swabs in the dryer to preserve evidence by preventing decomposition from moisture.

I removed my gloves. "I'm finished with this part of the procedure, Jamie. Do you have any questions?"

The young girl uncovered her face. "No. I just want to be done."

Shannon held up the tweezers. "I saved the worst till last."

Jamie snapped her knees together. "You ain't doin' it."

Shannon stepped back to give Jamie space. "You need to reconsider if you want the guy in jail. Think about it. How about pulling a few sample hairs out yourself?"

Jamie winced at the thought, but after a few moments, she agreed. "I'll do it. Just tell me how many." She yanked and counted each one, placing them in an envelope.

Shannon drew blood samples to test for syphilis, hepatitis, and HIV. She checked off items on the collection list. "What prophylactic antibiotics do you want to give her?"

Jamie sat straight up. "No shots."

"Could you swallow several pills?"

"Sure. I'm good at pills." Her lips smiled, but her eyes remained cold. "I drop a lotta drugs, but I'm not an addict."

I left the room to dictate and ordered Jamie's medication. When I was headed back to the room with the meds, I found Detective Jones waiting near the door. "Hey Kelly, are you finished with Jamie? I need to talk to her."

"She's getting dressed. It will be a few minutes before she's ready. Let me give these to her, then I'll tell you what I know about her situation." I handed the pills to Shannon.

Cy and I walked back to the dictation office. "Do you have any more information on the stab victim?"

"The 911 call came from a cell phone in the vicinity. I'm hoping we can trace it."

"Too bad you had to come back twice in one night. I didn't see you at all last week. Where were you?"

"In Oregon. I spent a week at the Coast. You should join me next time at Cannon Beach."

"I don't get much time off, but if you're serious, call me when you're going again."

"I'm serious, but you have to like dogs. I don't go anywhere without Jax, my black German Shepherd. He retired from the canine unit after a leg injury."

"I love dogs. Is his leg okay?"

"He's finally walking on it after surgery. Do you have time for a cup of coffee?"

"I don't. Morning report will begin soon and I need sleep."

"At least your hair had time to dry since my last visit." His eyes lit up with his smile.

Cy always brightened my spirits, but he'd never invited me out before. "I need to finish this residency before it finishes me!"

"You need to study playing now and then instead of always doing medicine." We sat down in the dictation cubicle.

"How's Jamie?"

"Good, under the circumstances. The poor kid would rather be on the streets than at home with her addict mother's latest boyfriend hitting on her. You don't have to turn her over to her mother, do you?"

"She's underage."

"I know, but she'll just run. Can't we get her into a safer situation?"

"I have to notify her mother."

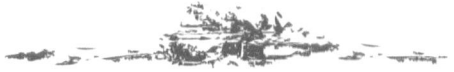

I went back to the room after my dictation and co-signed the evidence collection forms with Shannon. She placed them inside the box, sealed it, and handed the evidence directly to Cy, completing the chain of custody. This process verified the kit was in our sight at all times until placed in police hands. Evidence tape sealed the brown paper bags containing Jamie's clothing, which was likely to contain trace evidence.

Later, Jamie waited near the exit for transportation to the shelter. She answered the detective's questions, and he authorized a safe-home placement. Showered and dressed in clothing donated to the ER for patients, she appeared slightly refreshed. "I hope you'll stay away from Broadway. Girls your age are being stabbed up there."

"I heard." Jamie looked at her feet. "I knew one of them." She started to say something but stopped mid-word and turned her back as Brett Warren approached. He lingered in the doorway of a nearby room looking at a chart and then entered out of earshot from us. Jamie whispered, "Who is he?"

"Dr. Warren, a surgeon."

Her ride arrived. Jamie mumbled, "Thanks." She cast another look at the doorway through which Brett had disappeared.

Automatic doors opened, allowing Jamie's escape.

I glimpsed the dull morning sky. Daylight brought the arrival of a fresh team of residents and medical students to join Dr. Hunter's dreaded critique of the preceding shift's activities. His interrogations, appropriately called the morning pyre, made most of us feel like we were being burned at the stake.

I tried to organize my thoughts so I could answer his probing questions.

Chapter 4 Competition

Dr. Hunter stood a head taller than most of the residents and medical students gathering around him for morning review. He always appeared more alert than most of us did after a full night's sleep. Hunter spoke with his eyes. They could be soft and blue or gunmetal with a steely stare piercing fear into the heart of a vulnerable understudy. Today, a blue shirt complemented his eyes, which were watching me approach the dozen staff members gathered around him. "Dr. McKay, I see you performed an emergency thoracotomy last night. Present your case first, your decision-making, and the outcome." He checked his watch. "You have two minutes."

I'd presented cases to Dr. Hunter for two and a half years, but he still intimidated me. I tried not to show my anxiety and addressed the group in a calm, deliberate way, explaining my reasons for opening the chest and the outcome.

Hunter's gentle eyes focused on each face in turn when I finished, then locked on mine. "If you don't try, if you're not aggressive enough or fast enough in decision-making, you'll lose lives." He held up the twenty-four-hour patient log. "It was seven minutes from ER arrival to incision."

Blank faces looked back in silence, not sure if he was pleased or angry because his tone had changed. "Group, that's fast. But you made a big mistake, McKay, a big mistake."

My face flushed and itchy blotches erupted on my neck which happens when I stressed. I knew where he was headed.

"Your blood exposure could kill you. Dr. Maddox was unforgivably careless." His steely eyes searched the group. "Where is she?" His tone angry, "I want to talk to both of you when we're done with critique."

The group buzzed in muted conversation.

I had seen her grab a chart and drag a medical student with her into a room to start on a patient evaluation. "She's here somewhere with a patient."

Hunter continued addressing the group. "Don't take this wrong. Dr. McKay made the right decision to open the chest. A few minutes ago, I checked with the medical examiner about the stabbing victim. He said no one could have saved her." Hunter searched the group and pointed. "And you, Dr. Warren, where were you when all this was happening?" Hunter didn't wait for an answer. "I'll talk to you later, too. Your failure to respond to a code is inexcusable. Let's go on to the next trauma case, your case, Dr. Warren." Hunter looked at a code report. "Why is it Dr. McKay opened a chest in about the same time it took you to get an airway in?"

Brett turned pale, his expression flat. He didn't respond.

"Dr. Warren, present this case. Tell us what you would do differently if you could start over." Hunter sounded professorial, but most of us knew how tough he could be and feared his barbs. Harsh criticism at the end of a long shift took a toll on self-esteem and the confidence of tired young physicians. Sometimes I found it difficult to explain my actions. This time, I waited for Brett's response.

He chose his words carefully. "This tough case has some teaching points. We were too slow placing a functional airway on a critical trauma victim." His voice trembled and then eased into a faster cadence. "I prepared to do a surgical airway but let anesthesia have one last try." He smiled. "We all learned from this case."

A convincing actor, he had recovered from his hesitant start.

Hunter aimed next at the anesthesiology resident. "How about you, Dr. Flora? You've been learning how to manage difficult airways for years. You'll be on your own in a few months. Where were your skills when this patient needed them?"

Milt's shoulders curved forward as if to protect his body and minimize injury. "I should have replaced the leaking tube over an exchanger. Bleeding from her floating facial fractures made oxygenation and intubation next to impossible, but I got it in."

Damn him for not giving the flight nurse credit for the intubation.

"Unfortunately, the patient will not survive, Dr. Flora, but it was not your ineptitude causing prolonged anoxia that will result in her death. I talked to the neurosurgeon, Neville Carrington. She has lethal brain trauma." Hunter addressed the group. "She's in ICU on life support, a POD, potential organ donor." Hunter eyed Milt and Brett. "It took both of you too long to get an airway. Totally unacceptable."

The gathered young physicians and students learned from these confrontational interrogations and knew they might be next.

"With facial injuries like hers, and blood in the airway, you cannot adequately mask ventilate. Anesthesia screwed up, but Warren, you were in charge." Hunter warned, "Don't let it happen again. You're a surgeon. For god's sake, cut! I'll fault you more for *not* doing a surgical airway than doing one when you had other options."

My good friend Lynn Cabot stood in the back, partially hidden from Hunter's view. She'd been up for the last twenty-four hours working like the rest of us, yet we'd barely spoken. We usually had coffee together, but the high ER volume had prevented socialization. Lynn listened to Hunter and smiled. Not many smiled at Hunter during morning reviews, but nothing fazed Lynn. In spite of the long shift, her wash-and-wear short blond hair looked perfect.

Brett paced, head down and tense, waiting to talk with Dr. Hunter about his failure to appear at the trauma code.

I talked with Hunter first. Concern furrowed his brow. "The rapid HIV screen on your addict patient was negative."

"I'm so glad. It was on my mind, but I didn't take time to call, probably because I dreaded hearing bad news." I breathed a sigh of relief and stretched my tense shoulders.

"As you know that test isn't foolproof. It could be a false negative. We'll get the final result in two days with the hepatitis screen." Hunter slammed down a clipboard. "I can't believe Mona did this to you!"

"I'm horrified, but at least she didn't cut a tendon. Maybe I was careless with my hand placement."

"No. It's not your fault, Kelly. Mona was the one with the scalpel." Hunter's tone changed from anger to sadness. "It's one of those things we wish we could do over. Backtrack. Rewind. I hope the tests for hepatitis are negative. Did you start treatment?"

"I took the initial three-drug dose a few hours ago. Before I leave for home, I'll pick up more at the pharmacy."

"I don't worry much with a contaminated needle stick because the conversion rate is so low. But after I reviewed this patient's drug history, I'd recommend you take prophylactic drugs even for a needle stick from her." Hunter pulled out a chair. "I think you should rest for a few minutes before driving home. You look very tired." His kind hand touched my shoulder. "Be sure you take triple drugs until we get final results, longer if there's any question."

I appreciated his concern, but it only increased my anxiety.

"The medications are nasty. They'll make you sick but could save your life." Concern in his voice emphasized the importance of his words. "Please don't stop taking them even if you feel terrible."

Mona hovered nearby talking with the medical students while eavesdropping on my conversation with Hunter. I split for the locker room, but as I walked away, I heard him say, "I'm shocked at your carelessness. What were you thinking, Dr. Maddox?"

I wanted to hang out and listen to Mona's excuses, but it would look too obvious, so I went to the locker room. Dressed in jeans and a purple sweatshirt with GO DAWGS emblazoned in gold, I faced the pharmacist. She handed me a bag of expensive medications to cover the next few days. She stressed the importance of continuing the pills no matter how bad they made me feel.

Acid seared my throat as I walked toward the exit. I doubted I could feel that bad after one dose and doubted I'd make it the five miles to my apartment on Eastlake Avenue without stopping to vomit. I dragged my feet across the ambulance entrance toward the parking garage. Lynn Cabot drove out in her red Porsche 928 and stopped. She lowered the window. "Kelly, I thought you'd like to know the students and the other docs gave you some compliments. This morning was one of Hunter's least painful reviews, don't you think?"

"It could have been worse."

"The med students groaned when I told them I'd be on a psychiatry rotation for a month and that Mona was back in ER."

"I feel the same way. Mona has a nasty habit of belittling everyone."

Lynn revved the rumbling engine. "Mona was talking with Hunter when I left. He was steaming."

I raised my bag of medications into her view.

"What's that?"

"The blood-exposure drugs. My gut hurts after one dose."

"Was the rapid HIV test negative?"

I nodded. "But knowing the patient's history and seeing her needle-tracked veins, I'm skeptical."

"I would be, too. Did Mona apologize?"

"No. She accused me of being clumsy and then offered to sew up my hand."

"I wouldn't let that bitch near me! Don't stop the drugs."

"I won't. I hope you enjoy your month on the locked ward."

Lynn frowned. "It won't be easy. They get the worst."

"I'd prefer psychiatry to working with Mona."

"She is too competitive, and her ugly attitude makes it worse. I heard her telling staff about showing up to help you in the nick of time." Lynn changed her voice to mimic Mona, 'The clown was up to her elbows in blood, inside a chest that never should have been opened.'"

"That bitch."

"You couldn't see her face from where you were standing, but she rolled her eyes and disagreed with Hunter's positive remarks about your skill."

"Sometimes I feel sorry for her, Lynn. She's so unhappy and unkempt. It looks like she chops her own hair off with a scalpel."

"Maybe she does. In any case, she gives lady docs a bad name."

"I shouldn't say anything. I probably don't look so good myself."

"You'll feel worse when you hear this. She's applying for the chief resident position."

"That's an ugly thought. She seems to hate it here."

"She's wicked. You'd better watch your back."

Chapter 5 A Job in July

Twenty-four hours off work never provided enough time away from ER responsibilities to do anything but sleep and eat. I had little time to review for the ER boards looming a few months after graduation. I learned a lot each day working with Dr. Hunter. Most of us thought of him as possessing vast RAM storage. When we asked him a question, he accessed his impressive databank. He always had the answer and a journal citation to support it, which set a high standard for the rest of us.

Dr. Hunter spent nearly as much time in ER as the residents and carried a pager, two radios, and a cell phone. He expected the same dedication from the residents. When off duty, he monitored ambulance radio calls and helicopter flight responses. Even in the middle of the night, from a bedside radio tuned to the emergency channel, he advised field medics responding to difficult calls. I wondered when he slept.

Medics described a helpful call from him one night when they were on scene with a child in cardiac arrest. Dr. Hunter's voice emanated from their radios like the voice of God giving them guidance.

Hunter supported medics and ER nurses with equal intensity. I witnessed his wrath against Milt Flora after he walked in on him castigating a nurse and a respiratory tech about an airway problem that Milt should have handled.

If a resident screwed up, Dr. Hunter assigned remedial work and verified that the young doctor followed through. His harsh demeanor mixed with his brilliance in teaching medicine blended with his empathy for patients. Years in the trenches of academia hadn't reduced his caring. He often reminded us in morning report of the honor it was to be a physician and ordered us to treat patients with respect at all times. We would disperse and begin caring for early arrivals that sometimes jarred my resolve to treat all patients with respect, especially those who verbally abused and spit on me. A common occurrence in the ER.

The shift twenty-four hours after my disastrous night began with a man complaining of severe back pain. I stood in the doorway out of view and observed his behavior.

The man sat in a contorted position on the edge of a chair. His pained expression and moans added to the theatrical scene. The distress appeared genuine until he dropped a pack of cigarettes that he snatched from the floor without a wince.

After a thorough exam and history, I gave him a prescription for physical therapy with instructions to follow up with a physician.

In the next dim room, an attractive young woman in tears sat hunched forward, hands over her eyes to block out light. She looked up when I entered. "Doctor, please help me. You look like such a nice woman. I know you'll understand." She pointed to her facial bruises. "My boyfriend beat me up yesterday." A ragged sob interrupted her story. "We made up, but this black eye really hurts. It gave me a killer migraine. I need something strong for pain. Demerol never works."

I turned on the lights and asked her questions about her headaches, head injuries and family history. She cried out periodically and covered her eyes during the thorough neurological exam. After checking her face and eyes and evaluating her reflexes, I opened an alcohol wipe and swiped across her cheek and around the "black eye."

She jerked and slapped my hand away. "That hurts. What are you doing?"

I showed her the alcohol wipe darkened by purplish makeup. "Do you want me to call the police or are you going to walk out of here right now and never come back again seeking drugs?"

She grabbed her large purse and brushed past me. "Bitch."

Mr. Back Pain waited for her. They had both failed to get narcotics from me. Her bruise makeup under dim lighting was very realistic. Brighter lights revealed flecks of sparkle in the dark tint used around her eye. Some days, ER beds filled with drug seekers using a myriad of creative complaints, but most of the time people with legitimate illnesses kept us busy. Without the triage nurse keeping ER traffic organized, physicians would have had difficulty knowing which patient to evaluate next.

A medical student stayed with me much of the shift as patients entered the ER in an endless stream. I supervised his exams and had him practice patient presentations. Sitting near each other repairing lacerations on two drunken men left over from the night shift, we discussed suturing technique. Our oblivious patients periodically trumpeted dueling snores.

"Dr. McKay, you're a lot easier to work with and learn from than Dr. Maddox. I feel so dumb around her."

I finished suturing and checked his work. "Mona acts the same way toward everyone, including me. She likes to push people's buttons." Closely spaced stitches on the gnarled old face pulled wound edges together into a perfect repair. "Good job. I think you'll grow up to be a plastic surgeon."

The student admired his work. "This was fun. You may be right."

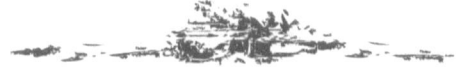

Harbor Medical Center ER treated close to two hundred patients every twenty-four hours. Physician-led teams ran to keep up. Regulars who could only get a ride at night, the naturally nocturnal creatures we called the "night owls," arrived in groups for care. Those with minor problems were "treated and streeted."

Most nights brought police officers and detectives to Harbor. Sometimes they just stopped for coffee. Cy Jones hadn't come in for days. I wanted to ask him about progress on the stabbing death cases he was investigating and asked Annie if she had any information. She hadn't seen him either.

Maybe no news is good news.

This night, five patients remained at 4 a.m. Two snoring drunks waited for detox evaluations. A psychotic man in leather restraints finally rested after receiving numerous calming drugs. His misfiring brain led him to believe the cars behind him on the freeway were following him, which, of course, they were. After he took evasive action and began driving erratically to avoid his pursuers, police pulled him over near the James Street freeway exit and brought him up the hill for an evaluation.

I admitted him to Psychiatry just before Hunter began a fiery interrogation of Mona about her comments to Brett after a teen death from a car accident. An unnamed medical student had had the courage to describe the scene privately to Dr. Hunter. The night had been easier than most for me, but for Mona, the confrontation with Hunter left her furious. In the physician lounge, she kicked a garbage can over and shoved a stack of magazines off a table to the floor. I stood near a locker changing clothes and watched her behavior in disgust. She stomped over to me and snarled in my face, "Did you tell Hunter what I said?"

"I was taking care of another trauma, but I heard about your inappropriate behavior from a number of people."

"Who? I want to know who. I'll kill the person who ratted to Hunter!"

"You won't get the chief job by acting out. Calm down and think before you speak."

"Don't tell me what to do."

I walked out and left her mumbling.

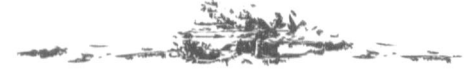

Aluminum foil taped to the windows of my bedroom allowed no light to enter and interrupt daylight sleeping. I took the HIV drugs and ate a container of yogurt to settle my stomach. When a phone call awakened me, the digital clock glowed green, 7:20. My thoughts did a rapid circuit. Morning or night? Am I late for work or can I sleep for ten hours?

I croaked a groggy hello and struggled to my feet. I flung open the bedroom door. Minimal light through the living room windows from a dark sky still didn't tell me the time of day.

"Hi, is that you, Kelly? It's Lynn."

"It's me. What's up?"

"It didn't sound like you. I thought you might want to go out to eat. A nice change from hospital food. Plus, I have to talk to you about a great idea, and no, I'm not selling Amway."

"I guess that means it's evening. From the way I felt when I answered and saw the time, I couldn't tell if I'd slept too little or overslept. Give me a minute to wake up. I'd love to join you."

"I'll pick you up. Wear something warm. It's cold and raining as usual. Don't go back to sleep."

"I won't. I'll be ready in half an hour."

I picked out some clothes to wear and then lit a cinnamon-scented jar candle in the living room. The flame cast flickering shadows across the walls. A warm glow filled the room. Its fragrance reminded me of home and my mother's apple pies. Nearly Christmas. I'd be away from home at Christmas for another year. I hadn't even bought gifts for my mother and sister. No time to shop. No energy. No holiday spirit.

While the coffee brewed, a shower shocked me to a higher level of alertness. I pulled on jeans, a green turtleneck, and an orange polar fleece sweater.

From my window high above Eastlake, the Lake Union skyline sparkled with street and traffic lights. Dark-roast Starbucks diluted with canned milk helped wake me up but burned my stomach after another dose of drugs. I felt better by the time Lynn knocked on the door.

"Kelly, I like the look! Orange hair, orange shirt. Good match. Are you ready to leave?"

"I'm ready and starving."

On the way to her car, Lynn said, "I think you're crazy to want that chief resident job. I don't think you should even apply. I've been thinking about next year and where to go when I finish in July. It's time to make a decision."

"I'm interested to hear about your plans. I may not get the chief position and will have to scramble to find a real job."

The red Porsche, a med school graduation gift from Lynn's parents, rumbled to life. "Where should we eat?"

"How about the Northlake Tavern for pizza and beer? We could bring home leftovers."

Lynn drove the short distance along Eastlake, crossed the Ship Canal, and turned beneath the bridge. Parking in Seattle was scarce, especially by the Northlake, but we found a place a block away. The line for seating extended outside the door and halfway down the street.

We finally made it inside for another wait. I enjoyed looking at the funny caricatures painted on the walls, and it gave us time to talk. Lynn announced, "I'm going to Alaska and I want you to come. I have jobs lined up for both of us."

I cringed. "I've always wanted to visit Alaska but have never thought of living there. Besides, I really want the chief resident job."

"You're nuts. Isn't eleven years of cutthroat competition in the university system long enough? On July first, I'm gone."

"Your mother will be apoplectic when she hears you're headed to Alaska."

"Mother talks about me *going into practice* and taking care of the society bitches, not her words exactly. She doesn't understand emergency medicine. To her, a broken fingernail is an emergency."

Our table against the wall in the back provided a quiet location to converse and eat. When we ordered two large pizzas, the waitress wanted to know, "How can two little women eat so much?"

Lynn explained. "We're bad cooks and love leftovers."

She wrote the order. "I've been known to drink warm coke and eat cold pizza myself, just like the Christine Lavin song."

I studied Lynn for a moment. "You used to talk about traveling to Europe."

"You can blame Annie. She has an ER doctor friend in Anchorage. I called him. I'm flying up next week for an interview."

"You're a city girl. What will you do with your Porsche in Alaska?" I pictured her driving that beautiful low-slung sports car over rutted dirt roads. "You'll need a pickup. You could leave your Porsche in Seattle for me." I coveted the flashy car.

"I might have to if you don't come along. I'll never go back East. It's too close to my controlling parents. If I'm lucky, they won't even visit me up in Anchorage."

"I'll be up to visit, for sure."

"Kelly, please come with me. Forget Seattle."

"I'll have to find a job somewhere if Mona gets the position. Alaska would be as good a place as any, but I can't plan that far ahead."

"We could go anywhere."

"I look at the chief resident job as another year of intensive training with Dr. Hunter. I'll learn much more from him when I'm not so stressed and tired."

"Maybe it's an escape from the real world. Can you take Hunter's heat for another year?" Lynn frowned. "If he has the final say, Mona won't get the job. That means your chances are good."

"Mona's strong competition. Very bright."

"Yeah, and she's an aggressive misfit. When Hunter's around, she's always trying to look good at someone else's expense." Lynn studied my bandaged hand as I brought a piece of pizza to my mouth. "I'm worried about your blood exposure. After my needle stick last year, I didn't sleep until I got the negative lab tests."

"I'm fretting about this patient's final results, but there's nothing more I can do. I'm taking HIV drugs and am covered for hep B with the immunization." I took another bite of spicy pizza laden with stringy hot cheese. "The drugs kill my stomach. The pizza tastes great but may come back to haunt me. All I ate this morning was yogurt."

Lynn rambled about the beauty and adventure of Alaska.

I tried to listen, but fear of HIV and aggressive forms of hepatitis surfed my thoughts and clouded Lynn's descriptions of her job possibility in Anchorage. After she dropped me back at my apartment, I ruminated about dying from AIDs.

Two pieces of pizza congealed in my stomach.

Chapter 6 One Thing after Another

We split from the morning report and headed to the main nursing desk for the triaged assignments. The charge nurse said, "Hurry if you can, Kelly. I have at least a dozen more with minor complaints in the waiting room." The radio interrupted her. A medic reported, "We are code three, five minutes out, with an overdose in respiratory distress from the Rosebrier."

The nurse turned back to me. "I'll have Lynn Cabot take the OD if you have some med students to help you with the six patients in rooms ready for treatment. Brett and Mona have the trauma in the first room that came in just before our shift started."

I finished my first patient and was dictating when the nurse stuck her head in. "I might need you. We have chaos in room 1. The teenager with head and chest injuries just died. Her family is in hysterics."

"That's terrible. Has the crisis team been called?"

"They are on the way. Mona added to the fray. I heard her say, 'You talk to the family. Just tell them the dumb die young.'"

"She's an uncaring bitch."

"Brett is trying to calm the family and Mona's back seeing patients."

My next patient in diabetic acidosis would take a while. I got started with a medical student when an overhead code blue page to ICU summoned the cardiac arrest team. ER docs couldn't respond but the assigned group included medical doctors, anesthesia, nurses, respiratory therapists, and a clinical pharmacist. The thundering herd of people trained in the latest resuscitation techniques and drugs ran to the ICU.

About an hour later, internal medicine resident Nick Ryan sat and put his head down on his arms. I wondered what was wrong. "Got a headache? This work could give you one."

Nick sat up slowly and leaned back. "No headache. We must have shocked that overdose thirty times before I gave up." He looked exhausted. "I left my wife last night and got stuck in traffic. It's been a bad day."

And I thought I felt bad. "I hope you can find a resolution."

Nick ran his fingers through his tousled hair. "It's difficult to have enough emotion left for a personal life when you've spent your day swimming with piranhas, but she doesn't get it." He clenched his fists. "Yesterday, I was fifteen minutes late for a breakfast party my wife had planned for her friends from the bank where she works. I'd been up all night and didn't want to go. She blew up at me later after I embarrassed her by falling asleep at the table." Nick stood up. "I need some coffee."

"People outside of medicine think our jobs are glamorous, like the television shows."

"Right. I'm staying with my parents and they're not sympathetic."

"We get so involved saving lives, we forget about living." I picked up the Dictaphone again, knowing I had to get back to work but hating to leave him. "We survive because we believe in delayed gratification, thinking how life will be better someday."

Nick said nothing.

"Wouldn't it be horrible if, when we're finally done, we still can't relax and have fun? Then we'll say, 'It'll be better when we retire. Just a few more years of this work and then we can play.'"

He groaned. "You should be a shrink."

I smiled. "Sleep does wonders for the psyche. Get caught up on sleep for a couple days and then take your wife out for a date."

"Thanks. Maybe we should transfer to Psychiatry where work hours are more tolerable."

"Hang on. We go to twelve-hour shifts in less than a month."

Mona's figure loomed in the doorway. "Cut the crap, Kelly. Get out here and help. You can't be doing book-length notes like medical residents when the drunks are calling to you." Mona scowled at Nick after insulting me.

I walked past her without a word.

Nick brushed past and left Mona standing alone.

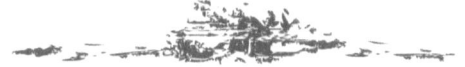

A couple of hours without a major trauma allowed the staff to clear out the waiting room. The charge nurse found me just after I discharged a patient. "Please come with me, Dr. McKay, we have a critical trauma patient arriving by air. It's not your turn, but I need to have you take this one. The others are still busy with a stabbing."

I followed her toward the main desk. "Their ETA is about ten minutes. Motorcycle versus truck. Multiple injuries, comatose, tubed, needled, on a backboard, and has two large IVs."

"Sounds like the medics have done a good job stabilizing him. I think I have time to start on one more patient before they arrive."

"Okay. Mona will be sorry to miss a good trauma. It's her turn, but she's with an unstable cardiac, a field arrest. Bystanders started CPR. Medics shocked him a few times and got a rhythm. He's in heart block. She's pacing him until the cardiac cath lab opens up."

Perfect. I'd love to take any patient just to rile Mona.

I listened to the final radio report at the desk and stepped outside beneath a dark sky to watch the touchdown and the usual drill. It always seemed we had more medical flights at night.

The helicopter landed and the crew off-loaded the patient onto the waiting gurney, and the jogging staff pulled the gurney toward me looking like a large running bug. The fight nurse held fast to the man's airway tube and squeezed the oxygen bag. "Hi, Doc. This motorcyclist slammed into a pickup at forty miles per hour. A witness said his bike hit a slick spot on the pavement." He took a deep breath. "On impact, the guy went airborne and landed on his head. No helmet."

ER doors opened. A blast of medicinal smells carried by escaping warm air brought a swirl of bad images through my thoughts, fuzzy recollections of emotional and physical pain during my rescue following plane crash injuries ten years earlier. Flashbacks happened at odd times and raised my heart rate. I gripped the stretcher and forced my thoughts back to the patient.

The flight medic went to the head of the stretcher to take over airway management as we entered the trauma room. His partner continued a barrage of information. The bright area looked like an operating-room theater. A dozen gowned staff members streamed in. Wall suction and oxygen ports, tubes, cardiac wires, overhead X-ray, all were ready for the unresponsive patient. Big-screen cardiac monitors blinked on standby, ready to record another patient disaster.

The trauma team members poised like a cast of players waiting in their places for the curtain to rise. They waited for the paramedic managing the airway to give the count. He was in charge of moving the patient from the stretcher to the ER bed. He alone ensured the airway wouldn't be yanked out by the transfer.

On the count of three, we lifted the backboard holding the man and moved him to the waiting bed.

The curtain rose.

The yellow-gowned team surrounded the bed performing their preordained jobs. Monitors displayed zigzag electrical heart tracings and flashed digital displays of blood pressure, heart rate, and blood oxygen saturation. Gone were the days when a nurse was assigned to manually pump up the blood pressure cuff and listen over an artery. Automated bedside vital signs had become the norm. The blood pressure cuff cycled, producing a running display on a screen.

A calm female anesthesia resident stood at the head working with the respiratory therapist, connecting a ventilator to the patient's tube. Soon, the automated machine cycled: inspiration, expiration, in, out.

The flight nurse continued his report as I examined the patient, and busy hands connected tubes and monitors, started another IV, and drew labs. "We tubed him at the scene. Skull fracture, fractured femur, chest, belly, and pelvic injuries. Has multiple rib fractures."

"You needled his chest?" I wanted to know their reasoning to warrant the invasive procedure.

"When we got there, he had no breath sounds on that side plus tracheal deviation. A palpable blood pressure at 60. After I decompressed his chest, his BP went from 60 to 80, and his trachea moved to midline."

I examined the location of the spaghetti-sized chest tube and listened to the patient's lungs. "Good placement. Fast work."

The medic reported, "He's on liters three and four of lactated Ringer's. Pupils have remained fixed and dilated. No light reaction at all."

I looked up into the faces of the disheveled flight nurse and paramedic as I listened to the injured chest. "He has unequal breath sounds, but I can hear some air movement on the right side. Great job, guys. He would have died without your quick work."

"Thanks. I'm not sure we're doing him any favors by the look of his head."

The team swarmed around the unconscious patient. Surgical resident Dr. Warren was nowhere to be seen. My voice harsh, I said, "Annie, where is Warren this time?"

The recording nurse heard my question and stat-paged Brett.

An oxygen saturation monitor clipped to the patient's finger showed 80 percent, maybe inaccurate because of blood vessel constriction in the limbs from shock. Metal leads stuck to his chest revealed a critical heart rate of 150. The low oxygen saturation, low blood pressure, and high heart rate set off alarms.

I ordered blood tests, transfusions, and X-rays.

A female medical student assigned to check for injury to the perineal area performed her exam. Like every examiner, she found doing a rectal exam on someone on a backboard no easy task. With help from other staff members, digging around between his legs, she announced, "No sign of scrotal, penile, or prostate injury." The sterile catheter she inserted produced grossly bloody urine from bladder or kidney trauma.

Organized chaos.

Noisy alarms, staff talking, suction noises, people scurrying, and no Dr. Warren. "We need a surgeon. Page Brett again."

Annie's scowl showed frustration. "I know his beeper isn't dead. I gave him new batteries tonight. We'll page him overhead again. We need OR on alert. He might be with them working on another case."

"Yes, and tell them we need a surgeon. This guy's in shock with a right-sided crush injury and may be bleeding internally from a liver laceration. We also need a neurosurgeon and an orthopedist."

Annie gave the recording nurse a string of orders without taking a break from her deft movements priming the rapid infuser with O negative blood. I heard the second page: "Dr. Brett Warren, Dr. Brett Warren, ER, stat."

A nurse announced, "The OR says trauma attending Dr. Lansing is doing surgery and can't come down. Warren isn't with them."

"Get the X-rays done. He needs a trauma CT, head to his knees if we can stabilize him." I reported my findings to the team. "His pupils are large and unreactive. He has subcutaneous air along the right chest, extending into the neck. Anyone who hasn't seen a patient with sub-Q air should feel this."

The med students followed my suggestion.

"With rib fractures and airway or lung injury, air escapes into the soft tissue. When you feel the skin, it crackles under your fingertips. Once you've felt it, you'll never forget." Two wide-eyed students behind protective goggles, with hands gloved and bodies covered with gowns, looked like the rest of us, afraid of contracting blood-borne diseases.

I clenched my fist and felt the stretch on my healing laceration, a grim reminder. "I need a size 32 chest tube. Pump in four units of O negative blood and keep me posted on response."

Smooth teamwork. X-rays, done. I listened to the lungs again. Reduced breath sounds on the patient's right side correlated with X-rays showing numerous rib fractures, a partially collapsed lung, and blood in the right chest cavity. His bruised, bloody chest crackled beneath my stethoscope.

I scrubbed an area of his chest free of blood in preparation for placing a large chest tube and uncovered a crude tattoo, the kind of artwork prisoners did on each other to pass the time. I cleared more blood and cocked my head to read the dark ink message smeared across his chest. It depicted a penis and balls with legs chasing a running vagina. The words beneath the picture read *Just one fucking thing after another.*

Team members strained to look at the tattoo. One respiratory therapist laughed out loud. His laugh stimulated others to look at the tattoo. Just then, Dr. Warren walked in, confused by the laughter in such a serious situation. His eyes went dark. "Kelly, I couldn't come after the first code page. I was talking to the parents of a dead teenager, and then I pronounced a DOA knife fighter."

"Tough job. So sorry."

Brett scanned the monitors and X-ray images. "What do you know so far?"

I gave him a quick report. "I think he's too unstable to risk taking him to CT. The surgery team will have to take him without imaging. I was just about to put in a chest tube. Do you want to do it?"

"Sure. Since you know the patient better than I do, I'll do the tube while you talk to the OR. We'll be ready to move him in five minutes." Brett looked around. "What was so funny when I walked in?" He walked to the X-ray monitors to examine the chest injury closer.

"You'll see when you place the tube."

Brett returned to the bedside and examined the man's chest. His eyes turned back to me and a faint smile crossed his sensuous lips. He cut through the tattooed balls and placed the tube.

Annie clasped the tube spewing bubbles and blood to a cell-saver suction that allowed the blood to be saved and filtered and then given back to the patient. "Blood pressure 90, heart rate 120."

Brett unlocked the bed wheels. "Get him on portable monitors and let's get to the OR before he crumps."

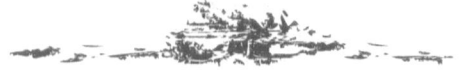

Dr. Lansing, attending trauma surgeon, met us in surgery and helped move the patient to an OR table. I detailed the injury incident, field interventions, patient exam, injuries, and X-ray findings.

"Thanks, Kelly. You got him to us fast." Lansing threw a disapproving look at Brett, "Where were you? Letting women do men's work? Why wasn't a neurosurgeon called to the ER? Maybe they should be drilling his skull while we look in his belly."

Chapter 7 Emotional Overload

Annie and I left Brett Warren in the OR with his surgical buddies. We rushed back toward the waiting throngs in the ER. Annie held the door to the stairwell. "Do you think he'll make it?"

"I doubt it. Even if they can stop the internal bleeding, his head injury, coupled with poor oxygenation from hemorrhagic shock, doesn't look good for brain function."

"I was talking about Dr. Warren. He'd been crying over that teenager who died. I've seen good doctors fail because of the stress around here."

I thought about his recent behavior and our interactions. "I don't know him well enough to comment. Seems nice. Sure is sexy."

"Brett isn't arrogant like Lansing, that bastard attending. Just remember, you're a better doctor than both of them put together."

"Thanks, Annie. I don't know Lansing and I try to ignore sexist remarks." We walked into ER. "There are so many male chauvinist pigs in medicine, after all these years I've become accustomed to their behavior."

"I haven't. Have you worked with Brett before?"

"Not until this rotation."

"Last year he threw a great party for the whole ER on his sailboat dockside at Shilshole Bay Marina. I don't remember seeing you there."

"I must have been working. I see a lot of tired, glum faces. We need something fun to look forward to.

"It was just before Christmas. The party did a lot to lighten things up. I'll ask him if he's going to do it again."

ER staff cheered when we entered. "Good job." Someone exclaimed, "We think you set a record getting him to the OR."

The cheer made me feel good, but Dr. Hunter didn't like the boisterous outburst. "Keep the cheering down. Patients will think we're having a party."

Two hours later, my beeper went off. I left a patient room and dialed the number. "This is Dr. McKay. I was paged."

A voice yelled, "Who paged McKay?"

The receiver crashed down. Repeated loud smacks reverberated. I pictured it dangling from a wire and slamming against the wall. The noise hurting my ear was replaced by a recognizable voice. "Hi, Miss Kelly, Russ Lansing. Sorry, my klutzy resident dropped the phone. Luckily, he didn't drop the scalpel. We saved your patient." Lansing sounded enthusiastic. "The guy had a lacerated liver and a small tear in the inferior vena cava. We packed his belly open. The bleeding is controlled, and he's in the tunnel of death with Neville Carrington for a brain CT scan."

Lansing covered the receiver and spoke to someone. He came back on line. "I just got a message from Carrington. The patient won't survive his brain injury. Carrington's going to talk to family members about organ donation. The liver was hamburger, so the transplant team won't want it. His kidneys should be good. Thought you'd want to know."

"Thanks for the update. Too bad."

The phone clicked. I felt terrible. The man had received the best of care and would still die.

Shannon stuck her head out of one of the private rooms at the end of the hall. Her tone urgent, she said, "Kelly, help me. Hurry! We're havin' a baby."

I ran to the room. A sterile pack containing a gown, drapes, towels, instruments, and a little rubber suction bulb lay open. A quick look between a screaming teenager's legs revealed a patch of wrinkly scalp with dark curly hair. The contraction eased and the head receded. With the next contraction, the teenage mother-to-be screeched, "I was raped! I was raped!" The girl's distraught mother grabbed her shoulder. "Who did this to you? You little slut. Your dad will kill you."

With the next push, the baby's grandmother dropped into the large chair by the bed and sobbed.

With Shannon's coaching, the teenager calmed down. After a few more pushes, a beautiful baby girl emerged and cried immediately. I suctioned her nose and mouth, then clamped and cut the cord. Shannon dried and wrapped the baby in a soft blanket. She handed the bundle to the new mother.

Instead of cuddling the newborn, the girl's hand shot out. She pushed the baby away and drew back as if frightened. "I'm givin' it up."

Shannon moved away, surprised by the young girl's reaction, and cradled the baby in her arms.

Grandmother stomped out of the room without looking at the baby or her daughter.

Mother rose up, resting on one elbow. She peered at the baby. "Is it black?"

I touched the wet curly hair. "The baby has light skin and beautiful dark hair."

"My racist parents hate my gorgeous boyfriend. He's part black. They made me stop seeing him. It's his baby." She held the sheet to her face and wiped a tear. "I couldn't tell him or them."

"That must have been difficult." I held the baby in my arms, admiring her beauty.

"I hid it from everyone. I even played volleyball and continued cheerleading. Then I sprained my ankle, so I had a reason to quit." She patted her flat belly. "Baggy clothes and being tall helped. I only gained ten pounds, but I took vitamins and drank lots of milk. I didn't want to deliver a freak."

"When did you tell your mother?"

"I wasn't going to tell her at all. I stayed home sick from school today. Pains started last night. This morning, after a gush of water, they got worse. I was going to drive myself to the hospital, but the pain got so bad I couldn't." Her thoughts were far away. "I called my mother at work and told her I had to go to the hospital. She had no clue. I should have taken a cab."

The teen's mother re-entered the room. "Get yourself together. We have to get home before your father does. Neither of us will survive his wrath if he ever finds out."

A nurse from the newborn nursery came in pushing an incubator. She reached for the baby.

An intense desire to keep her swept over me. I whispered to the nurse, "How could they give her up? Just give her away?" I took hold of her tiny hand.

Miniature fingers curled around my finger and held tight. Her eyes squinted in the bright lights.

The nurse studied my face, then the baby's hand. "It happens all the time."

Tears welled in my eyes. I held the tiny girl as long as I could.

The baby whimpered when the nurse took her from me.

I turned back to the teen mom and delivered the placenta.

She refused admission to the hospital, signed out against medical advice, and left with her mother.

I escaped to the far end of the hall and sat on a chair, trying to hold back tears. That beautiful baby, alone. No one to love and care for her. Thrown away.

A firm hand squeezed my shoulder. I looked up to find Brett Warren.

Tears spilled down my cheeks. I swallowed. A sob stuck in my throat. I couldn't speak.

"Kelly, it's okay to cry. Around here we keep everything inside." He looked into my face, "You're beautiful when you cry."

I had no words. I hated being seen weeping. Besides, I didn't know him. I mumbled, "Thanks."

Brett took my hand and squeezed it just for a moment and then disappeared.

Maybe my emotional wall was cracking under the strain of long hours and intimate contact with the unending troubles of humanity. Crying over the baby when I hadn't cried in years left me wondering. Why now? I'd hidden my feelings since the plane crash when my dad died and mother blamed me for his death. I thought I'd buried those feelings, and it made me furious to have lost control.

To survive in this business, you have to suppress feelings, even if it's unhealthy. I've never been one to discuss fears or problems with anyone. I consider it a sign of weakness, and I detest weakness. But experiencing Brett's tenderness felt good. It placed him in a different light. He'd treated some rough cases recently, and it had taken a toll on his emotions, too.

The remaining hours passed with only a glimpse of Brett. As I headed out the door on my way home in the morning, I caught the flash of a smile when our eyes met. A warm, unsettling feeling enveloped me. Too many emotions to process, and those damn HIV meds were tearing at my stomach. From the way I felt, I could have wondered if I had morning sickness, but in my case it would have to be an immaculate conception.

Before going home, I went to the lab to check my blood results. I'd lost weight. My stomach hurt so much that in the past twenty-four hours I'd only eaten one container of yogurt.

"Results on the source patient are not back, Dr. Mc Kay, but the HIV is here." The tech printed out the result and handed it to me. She stood still and watched me.

I felt faint as I scanned for the values. "What a relief. Thanks. Now I can stop those awful drugs." I returned to ER and told Hunter.

Relief eased his scowl. A rare touch of his hand on my arm added to his sincerity. "I couldn't be happier. Now, go home and have a good day's sleep."

I wanted to soar, rent an airplane, decompress, and celebrate by flying, but first, sleep. I was too tired to go flying or to call anyone.

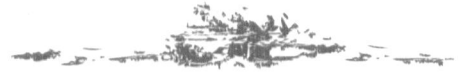

Afternoon darkness had fallen by the time I awakened, too tired to do much of anything. I decided to call my good friend and neurology resident Jen Markus. We didn't cross paths often, and I wanted to say hello. I had my hand on the phone when a ring startled me.

"Hey, Kelly, this is Brett Warren." My heart rate spiked. "I hope you don't mind me calling. I didn't want to awaken you, but thought you might be awake about now if you sleep as soon as you get off shift like I do."

"Nice to hear from you. I just got up, but I'm not really awake." I hoped I didn't sound too eager.

"Could I entice you to join me for dinner tonight?"

"Sounds great."

"Is there a nice restaurant you'd like to try?"

"I like the Thai restaurant on Eastlake not far from here. They serve great food in a quiet atmosphere." I should eat oatmeal, based on my stomach just one day off HIV drugs. We agreed on a time and I gave him directions to my apartment. "Come in on the alley. It's the only way into my apartment other than through the garage. The building's on a steep hill."

He laughed. "You're not in Kansas anymore."

"Right, but in Seattle the architects really have to be creative. My apartment is technically on the third floor on the front side, and ground level from the back. Just park in the alley. I'll be ready."

I dialed Jen and then Lynn. Neither were home. I left the great news about the negative blood tests ending the drugs and about my date. A hot shower and quick transition into black velvet leggings topped by a long teal mohair sweater, a touch of makeup, Shalimar perfume, and I was ready. I felt anxious but more rested and cheerful than I had in days.

It had been a long time since I'd been on a date.

Unlike at work, Brett arrived on time, bright and cheery, "Nice seeing you outside the ER."

"It's good to do something fun. Come in. I'll grab a coat."

Brett stepped inside and looked around. "You might need an umbrella. It's raining again."

I smiled. "I'm told real Seattleites don't use umbrellas." I pulled on a hooded coat.

"It usually doesn't rain hard enough to put up with the hassle of carrying one."

We stepped out into a typical Seattle mist and made our way along the mossy path to his car.

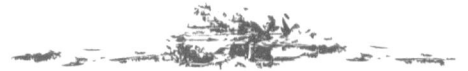

The elegance of dark wood, linen tablecloths, candles, and soft music added to the ambience in the dark corner where the hostess seated us. I'd eaten there before with Jen and Lynn. We'd enjoyed the food, but tonight I would have been happy eating hot dogs sitting in the rain next to Brett.

When he placed an arm around my shoulders, I smelled the same faint cologne I'd sensed when his face touched mine over a patient exam. His hand on my shoulder in the dark CT suite had stimulated the same irresistible pull I felt tonight, leaning against him reading the wine menu.

He ordered Tempranillo from a local winery. The dark wine relaxed my self-consciousness making it easier to converse. We talked about decisions that brought us to the University of Washington teaching hospitals and ways to combat the stress of our professions. For me, the topic segued to flying. I decided not to tell him about the crash that had killed my father and nearly killed me. Few people understood how I could fly after that experience.

Brett relaxed against the leather booth sipping his wine. "Can't say I'd find flying relaxing, but even when I don't have time to sail, I go down to Shilshole and stay on my boat. The gentle rocking puts me to sleep."

"I grew up on Minnesota lakes with lapping waves and the eerie calls of loons, but have had little experience sailing."

During the delicious meal, our conversation topics strayed far from medicine and surgery ending with an invitation to go sailing with him. His eyes opened wide in fake fear when I invited him to go flying.

"Promise, I won't do loops and rolls on your first flight."

He laughed. "I might need a barf bag if you do."

We talked with ease en route back to my apartment. His frowns at work had changed to smiles. I didn't want the night to end, but feared I'd fall asleep mid-sentence if I invited him inside.

When walking me to the door, Brett acted silly, maybe a little drunk, holding hands and swinging my arm like a kid. I stepped up one step and turned to face him. Light rain tickled my face as we melted into a sensuous kiss that ended leaving me breathless.

Brett held me at arm's length and smiled. His eyes turned feral. "I better leave. You have special powers, Kelly."

I wiped the mist from his face and kissed him softly, wanting to pull him inside, surprised at the desire he'd produced in those few moments.

He took the keys from my hand and unlocked the door. "I'll call you Sunday to go sailing." His lips brushed mine again. "Sleep well, Kelly, I'll be thinking of you."

I waved when he drove off and leaned against the door waiting for the passion to pass.

Chapter 8 An Escape

Brett talked to me only about shared patients in the days following our date. He walked away from friendly conversations with others. No casual conversation. I felt a sense of avoidance. His behavior left me confused, but on Sunday morning at the end of our 24-hour ER shift, he caught up with me outside the ER as I walked to the parking garage. "You haven't forgotten about going sailing later today, have you?"

I assured him I hadn't forgotten.

His call awakened me about 2 p.m. "You sound like you could use some coffee. Did you get some sleep?"

"Five hours. I feel pretty good."

"I'll be there soon. We can't waste time on a beautiful sunny Seattle day."

By the time the doorbell rang, I had showered and just finished dressing. A male voice called out, "Coffee delivery for Dr. McKay."

Brett handed me a latte. "Thanks for coming. It should be a great day out on the water."

"It sounds wonderful, but the only sailing I've done is a Hobie Cat on a small Minnesota lake."

"Puget Sound salt water can be challenging, but I usually sail alone. It's cold out on the open water in December, so you'll need a warm hooded jacket."

I placed my coffee on a table and pulled a ski jacket from the back of my closet.

"Perfect. That will keep you warm."

I took another sip. "The coffee tastes good. Thanks for bringing it."

"I picked up some bagels, cream cheese, and smoked salmon for lunch on the boat."

"Super." I tugged a yellow polar fleece over my head and was about to pick up my coffee to leave when swept me into a Starbucks-flavored kiss. His green eyes added a hypnotic effect leaving me weak.

"It's good to see you away from the hospital, Kel. You look great in scrubs, but it's nice to see you wearing something different . . . or maybe nothing." He raised his eyebrows and smiled.

I flushed and hoped he didn't notice.

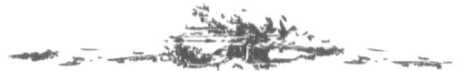

The drive to Shilshole Bay Marina took us down the steep grade past the Golden Gardens beachfront park. Rainbow sails of racing boats dotted Puget Sound, challenging each other on the sparkling water. Brett's warm hand on my knee generated thoughts of a wonderful day together. He pointed to the boats. "We'll join them soon."

The barnacle-encrusted pier of Dock C held the *Chippie* secure in a gentle breeze carrying the coastal odors of fish and seaweed. The white sailboat with polished dark wood trim rocked on the sheltered tidal water. Her lines lay coiled in artistic spirals on the deck. Brett untied the boat and boarded, then offered me a hand to help me step on.

We motored away from the dock and idled while he pulled up bumpers, then turned toward the breakwater past bellowing sea lions gathered on the rocks. They barked ferocious warnings as we passed and entered open water.

Brett raised and set the sails, pulling the lines and wrapping them with surgical precision around cleats.

A brisk wind from the south pushed us north. Three dolphins followed for a distance, dipping and playing before disappearing. Once clear of the sailboat race, Brett engaged the autopilot and disappeared below deck. He returned a few minutes later with two ski hats under one arm, juggling hot buttered rum in thermal cups and a lunch bag.

We sat on the aft deck on the cold breezy day, warmed by our clothing and hot, delicious drinks. I felt warm inside and out as we sailed in silence. Water slapped the hull. We watched passing luxury yachts, ferries, and ocean-going freighters as we skimmed along with the wind at our backs. Brett's apparent comfort sailing on the open water of Puget Sound gave me confidence in his skills.

We talked little about the hospital. I listened to him talk about the boat. "At twenty-eight feet, she's easy to sail alone. I stay in port when it's too nasty and work on the teak. It keeps me busy sanding and oiling." Brett sat leaned back with his eyes closed. After a few minutes of silence, I thought he might have fallen asleep.

I didn't dare close my eyes. I sat alert, knowing the autopilot was carrying us along a set route. I worried about hitting another boat or getting in the way of a large ship or a tugboat pulling a barge.

Short pieces of yarn attached to the leading edge of the sail fluttered in the wind. I wondered what they were for but didn't want to disturb Brett.

A feeling of peacefulness, away from city traffic and crowds, silent but for sloshing waves and a few seagull cries, swept me far from the tribulations of work. Happy people waved from a ferry.

Fleeting thoughts of the homicide victim found their way into my consciousness. I wondered if the detectives had made any progress in finding the murderer. Brett stirred and brought me back to sailing. I said, "You look relaxed and at home on the water."

"I am. I sailed on this boat for years with my Uncle Harry. He died of lung cancer two years ago and left the boat to me."

"I'm sorry you lost his companionship. He must have known you loved the boat."

"He did. He taught me everything I know about sailing and a lot more. Harry was more of a dad than his brother, my alcoholic father."

"You're lucky to have had such a great relationship.

"Thirty years as a Seattle police officer made him appreciate time off. He and his wife loved to sail."

The icy peak of Mount Baker rose taller in the sky as the wind pushed us north. Powerful sea-going tugs towing heavily loaded barges passed us periodically, sending our small craft rocking.

"After she died, Harry never looked at another woman. His only loves were his wife and the sailboat he named *Chippie*, his mistress."

"Wouldn't it be nice if our lives were that simple?"

"I look forward to that day." Brett fiddled with his marine GPS and changed the direction of the *Chippie*'s autopilot. The marine instrument gave him our position and speed over the bottom. Sonar fed us depth information. Modern technology kept us on course, simplifying sailing while we were distracted by our new relationship. "I almost live on my sailboat. It's calming when the rest of the world is crazy."

Sailing showed me there could be peace and life outside of medicine. A sudden noise startled me. Water turbulence sent us pitching in the wake of a large container vessel passing close by in the shipping lane.

Brett checked the time. "We'd better turn south so we can make it back before dark."

The wind died down, forcing us to motor most of the way to the marina. I stood at the stern and looked at other boats docked near us. A duck paddled by. A blue heron posed like a statue as it fished on another dock across the waterway. Sparse clouds were edged with silver against an orange sky, and there were painted reflections on the dark salt water.

Brett wrapped his arms around me. "Pretty sky. Pretty lady." He smiled and gently kissed my lips. I'd had few relationships, but no other male had ever had such a powerful effect on me. Brett left me distracted by desire and an uneasy sense of loss of control.

The sun dropped out of view, leaving us in semidarkness until pier lights came on and illuminated the area. Brett led me down the ladder into the hold. A small galley was on the left. On the right, a map table with an elevated chair. Polished teak covered the inside hull. A narrow shelf with a dark wood railing held a library of books on tides, fishing, and navigation.

Wrapped in a purple and gold UW blanket, I snuggled on the oval couch watching Brett in the galley. A kerosene lantern over the table swung as the boat rocked, splashing shadows up and down, up and down in a hypnotizing dance.

Brett caught me fixated on the lantern. "Do you have a fascination with fire?"

"Not anymore. I try to avoid it."

Steam rising from a copper kettle on a blue flame fogged the small windows. He poured hot water in cups for our rum drinks and brought them to the table. Sitting close, leaning against me, his long legs stretched out beneath the table. "I want to stay here and never go back to work. Surgery is killing me." He sipped his drink. "I'm considering quitting my residency."

I sat straight up. "You can't mean that! We all have bad days."

"After enough sleep and an escape on the water, I feel more positive, but not much. It's getting worse."

"You can escape to this haven and unwind."

"You're right, but some days I wonder why I ever thought I wanted to become a surgeon."

"I think we're both examples of cumulative stress. Burnout. A few days ago, I was thinking about going into law enforcement."

Brett laughed. "You don't look like the cop type. Besides, you're a very good ER doctor and only have six months left. You can stick it out. I have two more years."

"I'm feeling much better than I did when we finished the shift this morning. Thank you for the wonderful day."

"It's not over. Are you hungry?"

"Starving."

"Me, too. I have the fixings for a chicken stir-fry with rice. Are you willing to try my cooking?"

"Sure, if you'll let me help."

"You can help by sitting there and talking to me. The galley is too small for two. Someday, I'd like to buy a 36-footer with more space and a real galley. Then, we could cook side-by-side."

Warm beneath the blanket, I could feel the rum flowing through my body.

"I like to cook. After Harry taught me some simple bachelor recipes, it was my job to cook when we sailed." Brett lit a jar candle. "We did overnighters in the San Juan Islands north of here. We often set out crab pots and fished."

The candle's flickering shadows blended with those from the lantern, crisscrossing against the dark wood. He placed steaming plates on the table. I swung my legs down beneath the table and sat up. He squeezed in next to me.

"Annie asked me about having a holiday dockside party for the ER. We had fun last year, but the group got too rowdy for this sedate dock. Stodgy liveaboards, here on Dock C, complained about the noise."

I ate voraciously in our warm hideaway filled with piano jazz from satellite radio. "We all could use a party. Maybe they'd behave better this year."

Devoid of stress.

A different world.

Brett placed our dishes on the counter and returned with vanilla ice cream topped with Grand Marnier liqueur. He sat down again and pressed against me, after releasing my barrette. Ringlets fell around my face. He twirled my hair with one hand while eating ice cream with the other.

I had trouble focusing on the delicious dessert, distracted by his touch.

He put his spoon down after a few bites. Then, he took my spoon from my hand and placed it on the table. Candlelight shadowed his sensuous lips, drawing me to him in a sweet liquor kiss, pulsating to my core.

My heart stumbled. "It must be the rum."

He shook his head. "I don't think so, Kelly." We kissed. Hands exploring, crushed together in the confines of the couch, with a table so close it didn't allow much room to move. "It's not rum, it's chemistry. I know it when I feel it. We have chemistry."

His gentle fingers traced the scars from my face down along my neck. Beneath my sweater, his warm hands caressed my back. I tensed, fearing a close relationship and the anguish of exposing my ugly burn scars. Alcohol and semidarkness helped soften my concerns.

"What happened to you, Kelly? These scars. It must have been painful."

My father and I crashed an airplane."

"You crashed?"

"I got my private pilot license before I got my driver's license."

"What happened?"

"Dad and I were returning from a scenic flight in his Cessna. A couple hundred feet above the ground, on landing, another plane clipped us. The other pilot didn't see us below him. His plane struck our tail section and destroyed Dad's ability to control the plane."

Brett squeezed my arm. "That sounds awful."

I hesitated and continued. "The impact nosed us over, crashing us into the trees near the dirt airstrip. A damaged wing tank dumped fuel and our plane caught fire."

"I'm surprised you survived." Brett hugged me. "I'm glad you did."

"Dad died. I could do nothing, and I still feel responsible for his death. Mother hated flying, but I would always go with him."

"It's not your fault. It's the asshole that hit you!"

"I know, but when mother sat in the burn unit with me, she said, 'Kelly, if you had refused to go, you wouldn't have these injuries and he'd be here today.' Her words made it worse." Maybe I was saying too much.

"Did your dad die instantly?"

"I think the impact crushed his chest. He gasped and asked me to take care of Mom and Kris before his eyes went blank. My gut knots at times when his face haunts me, in flashes, in dreams."

"It was an accident. Not your fault." Brett's arm tightened around my shoulders.

"Nothing would have helped him, but I think that's why I'm in medicine, still trying to save him."

"How can you stand to fly?"

"I forced myself to fly as soon as the cast was off my leg. Like getting back on the horse that bucked you off. One of Dad's best friends went with me."

"I can't believe you'd do that to yourself."

"I had to get over it. I awakened night after night in the burn unit smelling smoke and screaming. When I tensed up on my first landing after the crash and flashed back, Dad's friend talked me through it." I laughed. "It wasn't funny then, but the dang guy made me do ten takeoffs and landings that day till some confidence returned."

"You owe him." Brett stroked my neck along the scars. "How did you get out of the plane?"

"I released my seatbelt but couldn't get the door open. I was stuck, screaming. Fuel streamed from a ruptured wing tank, and in a poof, the fire started." I took a bite of my melting ice cream to cool my throat and nerves from talking about the crash scene. "People were yelling and jerking on the door. The men dragged me away from the burning plane and smothered the flames."

His fingers on my scar triggered an irritation, too much, too close, and the desire to run surged. My panic built. I held his fingers to stop the touch and took a deep breath.

"Don't worry about the scars. We all have scars. You're beautiful, but maybe a little crazy because you actually still like to fly." He got up and went to the galley, where he poured two small glasses of Grand Marnier.

I looked forward to the liqueur's sedation to dull the brewing panic.

Brett pulled me forward toward the V-berth.

I had to control the rising panic. The V-berth looked small. Claustrophobic. I hated small spaces.

Brett handed me both drinks. I held them while he climbed onto the soft bed that had colorful soft pillows placed along the hull. He turned the comforter back and took the drinks from me. I followed him and sat against a pillow.

We sipped.

We talked.

We kissed.

My panic ebbed.

Brett seemed to accept me with all my baggage. He finished his drink and pulled me into a kiss, loosening my jeans.

I slid them off and removed my shirt, leaving my lacy underwear and bra.

He caressed my abdomen, my shoulders, my breasts.

Dim light from the dock through small windows in the bow gave me a shadowy view as he stripped off his shirt.

I ached, watching him loosen his jeans and slip them off. I held my breath.

In the shadows, Brett turned to his side. Our bodies melted together. His hands explored. Sounds of the water. The wind moaning in the wires joined mine. His caresses aroused feelings I had not allowed myself to experience with anyone before. He removed my bra and nuzzled the scarred right breast.

Barriers to intimacy dissolved.

Enveloped in a down cocoon, in his control, my life changed. Away from a chaotic world, he brought me with him to an addictive, emotional summation of desire . . . and then sleep.

Chapter 9 Party Time

Brett's dock party materialized a week later on an overcast December Saturday afternoon. Happy voices carried to the street level along the floating moorage and up the Dock C walkway. Laughter mixed with the familiar screams of seagulls announcing their presence while scavenging shore debris and tidbits from partiers. A couple of dozen people dressed in colorful windbreakers sat on the boat and along the dock. The setting could have been a photo shoot for a sportswear ad.

One of the nurses saw me on the steep gangplank making my way to the steel security gate protecting an expensive array of watercraft lining the moorage. She opened the gate. "Kelly, I hope our friends can navigate this route to the shore side bathroom after a few glasses of cheer."

"They better not fall in the water. I'm not in the mood to do mouth-to-mouth on anyone."

She pointed. "Unless it's that cute med student stud over there."

Brett called to me from the boat. Handsome in his fisherman's-knit sweater over a green turtleneck, he appeared relaxed or drunk, as did the rest of the group, talking and laughing a little too loudly. "Hi, Kelly." He held out a tray of cheese and crackers. "Are you hungry?"

"Always." But for more than cheese. I smiled and took a sampling. "Thanks."

Brett gestured, "That cooler by the helm is filled with beer or, if you prefer wine, I have some cups and a great box wine in the cooler." He held out a hand to me as I stepped onto the boat.

I filled a cup with white wine. Brett walked to the bow. "Welcome, everyone. Glad you could come to the second annual pre-holiday dock party. The head on the boat is too small to accommodate a party this size. I'd like you to use the public restrooms at the top of the ramp to the left. Some people live on boats moored here, so we need to keep the noise down to a dull roar. Have a good time and don't fall in."

The group cheered. The gate opened and clanged shut repeatedly for trips up and down the walkway and for newcomers. Annie joined me in the aft deck seating area. We sipped wine and listened to descriptions of life-and-death achievements performed by the male physician contingent conversing near us. "Those guys remind me of stories I heard when I hunted with my dad and his friends back in Minnesota."

"I know what you mean, Kelly. I suppose it's okay for them to share their stories here where non-medical people won't hear them. The discussions might save a life someday."

"If outsiders heard them, they might be horrified by some of the details." I looked around at the crowd and spotted the surgery resident we called Howie the Knife dressed in high-water pants and white socks. He didn't pay the slightest attention to the conversations of interns and residents proclaiming their medical feats. Howie's attention focused solely on Shannon, the new attractive RN.

"Most of the world has no clue what we deal with every day. Medicine isn't home visits and handholding anymore." I stood and looked westward at the beautiful boats moored across from us. "Many patients we see are demanding and lawsuit-happy, looking for a big win in the malpractice lottery."

Annie reminded me, "And patients carry fatal diseases. In the ER, our risks are so high. I'm sure glad that murder victim's blood came back negative for HIV and hepatitis."

"I lucked out. I don't like the exposure risks, but I love ER and medicine." I passed the cheese plate to Annie. "Medicine's a competitive, male-dominated profession, but I think that part is improving."

"Fifteen years ago when I started working at Harbor Medical Center as a nurse, there were very few women in medical school." She surveyed the group. "There still aren't enough."

I placed the hors d'oeuvres platter back near the wine. Someone squeezed in close behind me. I felt an arm around my shoulder, and the hand slid down to my lower back and then my butt. I thought it was Brett and leaned toward him.

Annie's look of surprise told me something else.

I turned. It was Neville Carrington. I detested the six-foot-tall, handsome neurosurgeon most of the female staff avoided. He made everything uncomfortably sexual. His fingers swished my hair. "Hi, Kelly, you beautiful woman. Isn't this a great party?"

"It is." I pulled away from him and sat down beside Annie for protection.

Annie elbowed me.

Neville didn't seem uncomfortable, even though neither of us made any effort to talk to him. Finally, he said, "What's new with you, McKay?"

"Not much," I said with disinterest. "Just glad July first is coming, even though I'm not sure what I'll be doing for the rest of my life."

"Have you talked to Lynn Cabot? She's leaving for Anchorage in July. Her interview went well last week and she got the job."

I was shocked to hear that news from him. "I talked to her over pizza last week, but her accepting the job is news to me." I shrugged. "I applied for the chief resident job or I'd go with her."

"I've read your application. You look great on paper, and even better in person." His eyes undressed me.

"Why would you be reading my application?"

"Hunter asked me to be on the interview panel."

"Is it a panel decision?"

Neville nodded. "The position's very important because the chief has to interface with all the attendings." He sat down next to me and sipped a beer. "Hunter wanted to be sure all the department heads agreed that they could work with the choice, someone we could trust."

"I'm anxious about the interview. I really want the job."

"You're hot, Kelly." His eyes lingered on my chest. "You have a better chance than the others. It's clear Hunter respects you."

"I get along well with him. I just hope the panel respects my skills."

Annie cut in. "Neville, for what it's worth, the ER staff and nurses love working with Kelly, the med students, too. We don't want Mona to get the position."

"There are others outside the University of Washington who have applied, but I think Kelly's application is the strongest." He drank the last of his beer and threw the cup in a trash can. "Lynn sure surprised me." His eyes were sad, downcast, "I can't see that city girl in the wilds of Alaska. I wish she wasn't leaving."

There must be something Lynn isn't telling me. I thought she'd dumped him a long time ago.

Neville zipped his jacket. "It's cold tonight. I hope you aren't sleeping alone, McKay." He smirked. "Let me know if you need any help getting the job."

Neville thanked Brett before he walked to the exit. The door clanged behind him. He slowly walked up the steep incline, alone.

Annie looked at me with disdain sweeping her face. "God, I dislike that man. He is such a womanizer. He makes my skin crawl."

"Slimy. Lynn went out with him a few times. I thought she'd lost her damn mind, but then she's always trying to help wounded birds."

"He is more of a vulture."

"I think it's been a year since she dumped him."

Darkness fell, along with a light rain. Complaints about noise from dock neighbors ended the party. Everyone left, and Brett had disappeared.

Annie helped me pick up cups and trash. We were about to leave when Brett stuck his head out of the hold. "Hey, Kelly, can you stay for a while?" He stepped up a couple of rungs and waved goodbye to Annie

I went down inside with him. "Great party. Thanks."

His words slurred. "Sorry I didn't get to talk to you much."

"You were busy playing host. I think everyone had a good time." He hung onto the table to steady himself. "It looks like you did, too."

We talked for a few minutes in the warmth of the boat. On deck, he'd be at risk of falling in the water since he couldn't walk without holding onto something. Brett sat on the couch and fell asleep mid sentence. I was glad he was inside and safe.

He toppled sideways on the oval couch, wedged in by the table, snoring. He was too tall to put his feet up, so I covered him with a blanket, checked the stove to be sure the burners were off, and blew out a lonely candle drowning itself in wax.

I made my way up to my car in the sparsely populated parking lot. A drenching rain added to my gloom and my disappointment that Brett had drunk to excess. I wondered if he'd been drinking hard liquor and hadn't realized how much.

We were not ending a joyous night together on his cozy boat. Our first sail together and great sex were etched into my brain. I wanted more of him, but after dealing with so many ER drunks, I was totally intolerant of the behavior.

Chapter 10 The Interview

Ruminating about Brett's drunkenness and the lack of an apologetic phone call during the next ER shift left me dejected and distracted. Our night together was nothing more than a tryst to him. So, why waste emotions on him when he didn't even have the courtesy to call? Mona Maddox's usual surly behavior sparked a few verbal exchanges, but Howie's enthusiasm for the difficult cases neutralized my negativity and made it easier to tolerate the Sunday ER traffic.

Working with Howie on a number of cases helped me understand Shannon's interest in him. His calm demeanor, combined with astute diagnostic and surgical skills, had earned him the apt nickname of Howie the Knife. The cheery guy wearing high-water scrub pants hiked up around his waist kept me smiling until the charge nurse walked up. "You're up for the next trauma, Kelly. Don't start a difficult patient until I see what happens. They just dispatched Medic 1 to a stabbing about three blocks from here. I might need you fast."

"Let me know as soon as you get a scene report."

The trauma alert ended in a non-transport DRT, dead right there. Medics came by later for coffee and told us it was another unfortunate drug addict, like the others.

The police had to stop the blood bath. I had to talk to Cy Jones. I hoped he'd find the killer soon. Hours later, he walked through the ambulance entrance and talked to Annie. She pointed my way.

"I thought you'd want to know, the killer struck again. This makes four."

"Horrible. You need a break?"

"I need to call the ME and could sure use a cup of coffee."

"We always have it on. I need some, too."

"Tonight, I'd even drink some of that tar you brew."

I led him back to the staff lounge, where he sank into the corner of a couch and pulled out his cell phone. I handed him a cup of fresh coffee as he talked to Dr. Del Ross. The county forensics lab was conveniently located in the basement of Harbor Medical Center. I'd interacted with Dr. Ross on a number of cases over the years and liked the skinny, professional man whose dry sense of humor often caught people off guard.

His face sober, eyes sad, Cy sipped silently for a few minutes, thinking and writing notes. "Dr. Ross is doing the autopsy on the last case this morning about eight. He'd like you to join us. He'd like you to see the findings on this victim, since you took care of the one earlier in the week."

I felt honored to be invited and chose to miss needed sleep to take advantage of the opportunity. Cy left to get a few hours of sleep before the autopsy. This was very bad timing for me since I had my chief resident interview in the afternoon.

A benign morning critique ended with Dr. Hunter wishing Mona and me luck in our afternoon interviews.

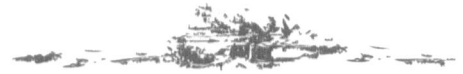

I took the stairs to the basement and buzzed for entry to the morgue. Dr. Ross, already in surgical scrubs and hat opened the door. "Welcome, Kelly. Cy's getting dressed. He should be out in a sec. You'll need scrubs, gown, double gloves. You know the routine."

Dr. Ross led us into the dissection lab where a body enclosed in a black bag lay on a stainless-steel table. He introduced a young man he called *Tim the diener*. "Tim and I took a look at her right after we got her this morning. All of these stabbing victims look similar." He unzipped the bag revealing a young white female in a black clothing with lips and eyebrows painted black.

Tim took multiple photos before weighing and measuring the body. After Ross examined her shirt and pants for particles, we helped remove the clothing. The diener took more photos before withdrawing vials of blood from a large femoral vessel. Then, he punctured her bladder, filling a syringe with dark yellow urine. "You want vitreous, too, Doc?"

Ross nodded and watched the young man extract fluid from the eyes.

Cy and I stood back and listened to Ross' explanation of their standard procedure. He flipped off the room lights to allow a thorough ultraviolet light exam like I used for ER rape exams. The special light illuminated semen, making it fluoresce in the darkness. Tim used moistened swabs to collect stains from areas near her pelvic area and around her mouth. He also took nail and hair samples.

Dr. Ross examined the left chest. "This stab looks different. It's bit angled and jagged, with another slash near it, not a single clean cut like the others. This victim is taller than the others, with a little more advantage, she might have been trying to fight off the assailant." He examined her skin front and back, then asked Tim to X-ray her chest.

We all stepped back to wait for him to finish. Cy filled us in on the investigation. "Four dead and we have no suspects. We put more plainclothesmen on the street in the Broadway District since all the victims have connections to the drug culture up there."

Dr. Ross asked, "Kelly, would you like to do the incision and give me and Tim a hand?"

My exhaustion didn't dim my interest in experiencing time with the respected forensic pathologist. He couldn't see my positive expression behind the mask, so I nodded. "Sure. What type of incision? The assistant handed me a scalpel.

"We have to save the tissue around the stab wound for microscopic evaluation, so for this one, I need a Y-incision beginning at each shoulder, meeting midline over the sternum at nipple level and extending to the pubis. Often, I do them angled beneath each breast but that puts the incision too close to this wound."

Once inside with chest tissue dissected and folded back, Tim sawed through the sternum. We opened the chest cage revealing lungs, heart and great vessels. Dark blood spilled from the gaping left side reminding me of my experience when Mona cut me. Seeing the gore and smelling death made my acid surge into my throat. I wished I was at home in bed sleeping but pushed on.

Dr. Ross handled the injured vessels with care, wiping the blood away to examine the cuts. "Findings are the same on all victims. Small external wound with mortal lacerations of chest vessels. I thought both of you would like to see this for yourselves." Cy and I looked inside the bloody cavity. His eyes drilled Cy. "The killer knows anatomy. These are precision stab wounds."

His words sent a chill through me.

Cy remained to talk. I thanked both of them and headed to the parking garage.

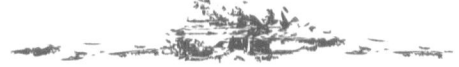

Stray sunbeams penetrated gray clouds. I had every intention of getting a few hours of sleep when I arrived home about eleven but ended up sitting in my recliner looking out over Lake Union, rehearsing questions the panel might ask. I watched floatplanes taking off and boats of all sizes trailing wakes on the dark water. Lynn Cabot's phone call startled me.

"I hope you weren't sleeping yet."

"No. Just got home after watching an autopsy on another murder victim. I'm finishing some oatmeal and thinking about the interview this afternoon."

"Neville said he'd be easy on you. I hope it goes well."

"Thanks." I took another bite. "I need encouragement."

Lynn sounded positive. "The attendings have worked with you for almost three years. Just be yourself."

"I wonder who else is being interviewed. Mona said one is a guy from Duke. His wife was accepted in a dermatology residency here."

"Just remember, Kelly, Anchorage could be a real adventure. We'd be flying all over Alaska if someone else gets the job."

"That sounds great, but aren't you too much of a city girl to like the wilds of Alaska?"

"On my trip up there, I loved it. My biggest achievement so far was leaving my socialite parents to come here. Alaska is my next challenge."

"Are you back with Neville? I was surprised when he brought up your name."

She sighed. "He needs a friend. I still like him."

Lynn always had men on her trail. When Neville Carrington first latched on, he took her on exotic dates, hot-air balloon rides, and romantic champagne dinners, but, much like her parents, he'd suffocated her.

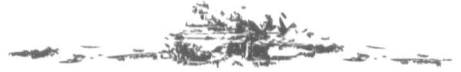

The interviews began at 2 p.m. After two hours of sleep, I arrived just before two and saw Mona's backside packed into a red power suit clear the doorway. She clomped into the room and down the aisle wearing three-inch heels, leaving two fidgety male applicants in her wake. I described the panel members to them and answered questions about the medical helicopter program and interdepartmental politics.

Mona emerged thirty minutes after her entry, cheeks and neck nearly as crimson as her suit, hands trembling. I'd never seen her so shaken, even under Hunter's fire. A trembling finger wiped perspiration from her upper lip. When she saw me, Mona screeched to a halt and gave me a once-over. "Kelly, why did you wear that ugly outfit? It's unflattering and certainly doesn't look professional." She stood tall and tugged her skirt down.

"I think they're more interested in what I have to say than how I look." I laughed. "Thanks for the compliment. You look very nice but not happy." She stomped off.

A passing medical resident overheard her comments and stopped to talk. "With somebody like her, you sure know where you stand. What are you two doing here?"

"Interviewing for chief resident."

"That explains it." He turned and watched her. "She doesn't like competition."

The door opened. "Dr. McKay."

The medical resident smiled. "Knock 'em dead."

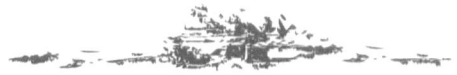

My beige slacks and satin apricot blouse felt just right. The pale color of the blouse complemented my reddish hair. At five feet two inches and 110 pounds, even in heels I didn't look old enough to the older attendings to even be a physician. At age twenty-nine, I had to convince the panel to let me teach medicine.

The door grated and clicked shut. The noise echoed in the large conference room, empty but for the panel of six men dressed in lab coats. The group sat around a large table situated on an elevated area one step up from the main floor. I looked from face to face as I walked down the long aisle toward them. Under the sting of their eyes, I felt like a model on a runway wearing see-through underwear.

My anxiety mounted. I wasn't sure where they wanted me to sit. Maybe the chair I chose would make a difference. Maybe that was part of their test. How does the candidate handle unknowns? Can she communicate? My thoughts flashed to a Charlie Brown cartoon from the past that pertained to me. Peppermint Patty was asked the numeric answer to a question on a math test. She answered "green." Patty had thought it was a trick question.

I tended to read things into questions too, making them harder than they really were. I hoped I didn't answer "green."

I stepped up to the table. "Hi. I'm looking forward to your questions." I nodded to Jackson Hunter, Surgical Attending Russ Lansing, and Neville Carrington. Six men greeted me. Neville stood and pulled out a chair for me at the end of the table near him.

Each department head asked questions in turn. Their flat expressions gave no hint of feedback or acknowledgment of my responses. They just waited for me to stop talking. Someone would ask, "Is that all?" If I said "Yes," then a question sounded from another panel member, such as, How do you handle stress? What are your interests other than medicine? Where do you see yourself in ten years? What's your greatest achievement? Why should we choose you?

I kept my answers light and short. I tried to remain calm and friendly. When they asked about other interests, I talked about flying and how experiencing serious injuries and burns had given me a special drive to do well in medicine and an understanding of people in crisis. I also focused on Lynn's words of encouragement, that the worst thing that could happen would be for them to choose someone else and then I'd be headed to Alaska.

The interrogation ended.

Before Dr. Hunter excused me, he said their decision would be announced after the holidays.

The session had lasted less than thirty minutes, and I walked toward the door feeling twelve eyes focused on my butt. Pompous men asking what sounded like benign questions made me uneasy. My future lay in their decision. I knew them well after working with them for more than two years. I'd seen them all make asses of themselves in front of groups. They already had my academic records. Maybe I should have given them longer answers.

Maybe I had answered "green."

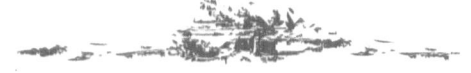

I walked out a hospital side door to avoid the chaos of the ER on my way toward the parking garage. Then, I remembered that Lynn was working on Psychiatry. I reversed course and took the elevator up to see if she had time to talk. I needed to clear my brain by doing something other than work or sleep. My nerves were shot and edging toward overload, with my surge protector about to fail.

Alone, enclosed in the elevator slowly rising to the locked psychiatric ward on the seventh floor, I felt claustrophobic, trapped in a burning plane. I couldn't breathe.

Floors 5 . . . 6 . . . 7.

My mental circuit breaker snapped.

I had to escape.

The doors opened and saved me.

I took a deep breath and walked out, trembling and furious at myself for my weakness. An hour with a massage therapist and a scenic flight would help, but I didn't have the time.

As I walked down a long hallway, my tension dissipated. I pushed the buzzer to gain entrance to the locked unit, thinking that maybe what I really needed a stint as a patient in the locked ward.

The orderly invited me in, which seemed ominous after my thoughts just before he answered the buzzer. I heard a scuffle and banging on walls, loud voices. I waited in the nursing station until Lynn freed herself from an agitated patient. She walked out of the patient room without a blonde curl out of place and beckoned me to follow her. "Let's talk in the hallway. It's too crazy in here right now.

The door clicked shut. "Well, how did the interview go?" Lynn gave me a hug.

"Okay, I think, but I'm wound up."

"You look good. Great outfit!"

"Thanks. Both Neville and Hunter were supportive, but it felt strange having a neurosurgeon on the selection panel."

Lynn defended Neville again. "He handles difficult ER cases and deals with the distraught families better than anyone else I've run across."

"I agree, but he's disgusting with all his sexual innuendos."

"Neville tries too hard. I have a surprise. He just told me he's inviting a bunch of us up to his island cabin over Memorial Day."

"Is he trying to cook up something just to be close to you?"

"I don't think so. His cabin is wonderful. It's small and isolated, located on an island with no ferry service. People can take a water taxi from the mainland." Lynn smiled and spread her arms wide. "I volunteered you to fly us up. There's an airstrip just down the hill from the cabin."

"I'd better get current flying if I'll be carrying passengers." Lynn had done a good job of distracting me. "We'll be four weeks from finishing the residency. That's something to celebrate!"

"Neville thought Memorial Day would be better than the July fourth holiday because too many of us will leave town at the end of June. If you get the chief job, you'll be working with the new residents then and wouldn't be able to join us."

"Do you know something I don't know?"

"No. I just think you're a natural choice."

"We'll know soon. Hunter said he'd announce their decision after January first."

The barred door opened into the hall. "Dr. Cabot, we need more sedatives for that guy. How about ten of Haldol?"

Lynn nodded. "Duty calls." The door closed, locking Lynn back inside with a madman.

Chapter 11 Confusion

Two anxiety-ridden hyperventilating women experiencing panic attacks began my shift. An entourage of family members and concerned boyfriends added to the turmoil. The patients didn't come in together and didn't know each other. Both believed they were dying and were in need of reassurance, but I had little comfort to offer. After the plane crash, I suffered similar panic episodes. I understood their mental haywire, but the distraction of mulling over my job interview blunted my empathy.

I worked in the same department with Brett for hours, sometimes side by side, before he disappeared. Not once did he speak to me except about patient issues. His professional behavior remained neutral, not unlike that of other team members. Brett still hadn't telephoned since the dock party. I had more than a casual interest in him after our earlier encounters and had hoped the feeling was mutual. It clearly wasn't.

Brett manipulated me and my feelings with such ease. I hated myself for allowing it to happen. He was sensational in bed and knew he had power over women.

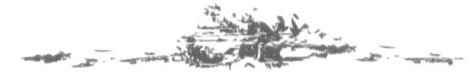

Annie leaned on a drunk patient, trying to hold his head still while I stitched his face. On his way home from the bar, he had pitched forward, splitting his forehead and lower lip. We ducked garlic-laden, alcohol-fumed profanities. I hummed and sang softly as I finished his forehead and then went to work stitching his lip. Hitting the moving target as he talked was no easy task.

Annie grasped his chin. "Kelly, you certainly sound like a little bird tonight. What's the occasion?"

I raised my voice so she could hear the melody and the words. "I've got the—I don't know what I want from you, Babe, but I ain't gettin' it—blues."

"I know that Ginny Reilly song. I sang it a few times myself before I married Carl. I dated a lot. Like most nurses, I made bad choices in men. When I met Carl, he said what he meant. No games. No surprises."

"Brett Warren and I went out a few times. He was great. I thought he liked me but he hasn't called. His behavior made me think of the song."

"I can see why."

"The song sums up my feelings. I must have misinterpreted his intentions."

"It's not you. He's a charmer but can change in a heartbeat. Be careful." Annie added, "One minute he's calm, the next he's verbally nasty and throwing things."

"I haven't seen that side."

"I hope you don't."

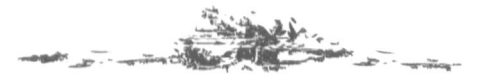

In the morning pyre, Hunter burned no one. He took me aside and said, "I'm pleased with your progress."

I left exhausted, burdened by ailing humanity and angered by no call from Brett Warren. En route home, I passed a few cars and entered the express lane. At home, I heard the phone ringing and rushed to unlock the door. Who would be calling at 8 a.m.?

"Brett, what a surprise to hear from you. I thought I must have offended you since you haven't talked to me since the party."

"No, you did nothing wrong. I'm ashamed of my behavior. I don't even remember half of the party."

"I didn't know what to think of your drunkenness and avoidance."

"I don't like the rumor mill at the hospital, so I try to keep things professional at work. I was concerned today when I saw you looking so sad."

"I've had a lot on my mind." He probably didn't care, anyway.

"Like what?"

"My job interview. Patients were getting to me, and I thought you were avoiding me."

"It's nothing like that, Kelly. When I should be thinking about surgery, I'm thinking about you."

I said nothing, doubting his truthfulness.

"You know how the staff talks about Neville Carrington. I don't want to be part of that grapevine. I like relationships private."

I made no comment.

"Could I come over to see you?"

"When?" In no mood to discuss issues while exhausted, I hoped he'd give me time to sleep.

"I'm still at the hospital. How about fifteen minutes?"

I was surprised by his request, thinking he'd ask me out. "I'm really tired, but come on over. I'm not in great shape and may not be the best company."

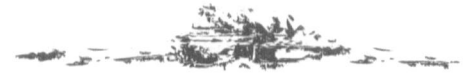

Before Brett tapped on my door lightly, as if trying not to disturb my neighbors, I'd slipped into a comfortable jogging outfit and brushed out my hair. I opened the door. Even in my exhausted state, I felt happy, and I melted when I saw his smiling face. After stewing about his avoidance behavior at work, seeing him brought a smile and a surge of emotion. I turned away. Damn, I hate it when I get teary.

Brett took my hand, led me into the bedroom, and swept me onto the bed. He lay beside me, holding me tight. He said nothing and was snoring in seconds.

I'd expected more, but I snuggled against his sensuous body and fell asleep. Later, we roused enough to slide beneath the warm covers and fall back asleep. Much later, I stirred to his warm hand caressing my breast, his body hard against mine. Enveloped in his arms, yielding to a sensational interlude of gentle love, my anxiety related to his perceived indifference faded. I drifted into a warm, floating sleep.

I awakened alone. He'd done it to me again! I felt used and abused. I had three hours left to sleep before joining the parade of cars on I-5 to reach the morning pyre. My stomach churned on empty.

I crawled out of bed and slipped into my jogging suit. On the kitchen counter, I found a note. *Kel, I slept well. Hope you feel rested and less worried about us. Brett.*

I felt worse because he'd sneaked out.

Canned tuna fish, tomato soup, and pasta; one of each remained on a shelf. Unfortunately, I mixed them all together. I knew it was a bad combination when the steamy smell wafted into the air. I ate one bowl and dumped the rest down the garbage disposal. The middle of a weird night was no time to experiment.

I'm such a bad cook, I'll eat most anything, but I'd finally found something too gross even for me. I turned to cereal, yogurt, and canned fruit.

The alarm at six awakened me enough to make my way to Harbor ER, where I dashed to the staff dressing room. Mona stood alone at the coffee pot filling a cup. I said, "Good morning."

She flipped her chopped-off hair and wafted a cloud of Red perfume. "Kelly, you'd better take that job in Alaska. Don't waste your time worrying about becoming chief resident. I've got it nailed."

"I wouldn't be so sure. We both have stiff competition."

"How do you know? Brown-nosing the attendings?"

"Hunter has obviously taken a formal approach to the selection. Some of the guys I talked with were from other programs. The panel is looking at medical capabilities, interpersonal skills, and academics."

Mona turned on her heel to leave. I called after her, "At least I'm still in the running. Your slash with the scalpel didn't give me HIV."

"Bully for you." The door closed behind her.

I put on a scrub suit and took a few minutes to call Lynn. I knew I could talk to her even though she wouldn't give me much encouragement about the job. I mentioned Mona's comments.

"Typical. She cuts no one any slack."

"She's trying to intimidate me. We've competed for years, but I've never felt such hostility."

"Don't let her bother you. You're lucky because I already have a job lined up for you if you aren't chosen."

I told her about Brett.

"I was hoping he wouldn't continue to complicate your life, but like most men, he is doing a fine job of it. Come to Alaska and marry a gold miner. Life would be so uncomplicated."

"I'm too inexperienced with men. I felt worse after he told me not to show any evidence of our relationship at work, as if he's ashamed of me."

"I don't know what to say except relationships shouldn't be complicated. Don't get too serious or you won't want to head north."

"I had hoped to know Brett better before he left for his next rotation. The last part of December he goes to the VA hospital."

"The VA will be easier for him than Harbor, but I doubt he'll get much time off."

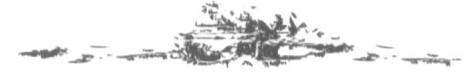

A week later, Brett caught up to me in the parking garage after morning report. "Kelly, hey, Kelly, wait for me. How can you walk so fast after being up all night?"

I stopped and waited for him. "I'm running to get to bed before I fall asleep on my feet."

"How about getting together later today after we both get some sleep?"

"I'd love it."

"Meet me at the boat about four?"

"Should I bring some wine?"

"Don't bring a thing. I'm going there now to sleep and will pick up something on my way that we can fix for dinner. Sleep well."

Mona drove out of the garage and laid on her horn as she passed us.

We stepped back.

Brett said, "That was unfriendly of her."

"That's Mona. She drives like a maniac."

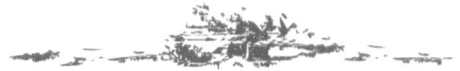

The alarm awakened me at three fifteen and I was out the door a few minutes later into light rain that became a downpour. Shaggy low clouds obscured my view over the salt water down the winding route to the marina, but it didn't dim my spirits. It had been way too long since Brett and I had been together on the boat.

I rattled the locked gate on Dock C. When I saw him inside, I called his name. The *Chippie* rocked as he walked to the ladder, emerging handsome, dressed in a gray jogging suit. He stepped off the boat to open the gate.

Brett held my arm on the slippery dock as I stepped onto the boat. When I descended the ladder into the hold, warmth and the smell of cinnamon wafted up to me.

"What would you like to sip, Kelly? I've just opened a Red Hook for myself."

"I'd better start with a Coke. It will help me wake up. I'll join you with a beer later."

Periodically, a gust rocked the boat and reminded us of the brewing storm. Mostly, the boat rocked gently as we sat at the table cradled by the soft couch. Luxurious pillows in each corner fit just right. The teak interior glowed richly in the soft light of an electric lamp hanging above the table. The cinnamon-scented jar candle flickered on the table in front of us.

"What kind of music do you want, Kelly? I could put on some CDs."

"How about classical or jazz?"

"I have a new Diana Krall piano jazz album. Let's see if you like it."

After I finished my Coke, Brett opened a Red Hook ale for me and popped open a can of peanuts. Periodically, a small heater beneath the table near my feet blasted warm air.

Brett leaned into his corner and spoke softly. "I love coming down here. When I'm by myself, I just lie in the V-berth and rock with the waves. It's like being in a womb, protected from everything bad."

"It's peaceful here."

"When I have trouble getting to sleep at my apartment, I drive down here. Wind in the shrouds sings an eerie tune and puts me to sleep almost immediately." Brett sipped his beer. "How are you holding up at work, Kelly? Have you heard if you got the job?"

"They won't announce a decision until January. I try not to think about it."

"I have two years left to complete the surgery program. Sometimes I don't think the struggle is worth it. If I had a different way to support myself, I'd quit now. I don't know how I'd tell my parents. They wouldn't understand."

His serious expression told me he meant what he said. "I wouldn't understand either. After all the years of work it has taken to get where you are, you need to stick it out." His eyes remained downcast, his expression like stone.

"Once you're in a swift current, it carries you along. You can't just stop." I felt like I was talking to a child. "You can't turn back. There are smooth, easy stretches, and then suddenly you're in a whitewater challenge." His unhappy eyes met mine. I added, "You ride it out, paddle harder."

He pulled back from me with a frown. "I've tried. I'm finding it harder every day."

"Hey, I'm done the end of June and figure I can stand anything till then, and you can, too." I hugged him.

"I think I'm in whitewater, caught in a whirlpool I can't escape." Brett slumped, head back on the pillow. "I've given up so much and am missing out on life. When was the last time you did things normal people do, like see a movie?"

"I can't remember. I used to read murder mysteries for fun, but lately I read medical texts. Most days are interesting but not fun."

"You're too studious."

"I really want the chief resident job. I've worked hard for the past two and a half years and tried to stay on Hunter's good side." Brett put his arm around me. "Actually, all through medical school I did my best, even graduated with honors. Someday I'll have time to play."

He pulled me to him. "I think we both need to play." A long look into his eyes sent a warm surge through my body, and I forgot what I had wanted to say.

Brett traced a vein on the back of my hand and up my arm as I took a sip of beer. "Nice IV site." He laughed. "Have you noticed how a career in medicine changes how we look at things, even veins?"

"I know. It's life changing."

"Tell me more about your family. There isn't much to tell about my family. I have an alcoholic father, a doting mother, and I'm a spoiled only child."

"It's just Mom, me, and my younger sister Kris since Dad died. He taught all of us to shoot, hunt and fish. He taught me to fly, and we shared that love. Mom hated flying. My scars remind me of his love and her hateful words. It's been ten years and we still aren't on very good terms."

"Your scars aren't bad, and your father left you with some good memories. My dad's a drunk who smokes like a fiend and should have died long ago. Instead, he hangs on and tortures my mother."

"Drinking takes a toll. My dad drank a beer now and then, but he had an alcoholic brother. I've seen what it can do to families."

"So, other than burns, did you have other crash injuries?"

"Open tib-fib fractures and a lumbar compression injury."

"For someone stuck in a burning airplane with those injuries, I'm surprised you survived."

"I was focused on Dad and didn't even realize my leg was broken. At first, a recurring image of his face and blank eyes followed me day and night. Even now, under some circumstances when a patient dies, a panic sweeps over me like when I watched him die." I stopped and thought. "I feel like I've failed once again when patients die. I should have done something more, studied harder, did it better."

"But Kelly, you can't dwell on that. He died from his injuries. You couldn't have saved him."

"Intellectually, I know that now. I'm a lot better than I used to be, but panic resurfaces once in a while."

"What about the burns? Somebody did a good job on you at the burn center."

"That part is a blur. I hate the scars but try to ignore them."

"Kelly, you're beautiful and smart. Remember that. We all have flaws."

I said nothing. He was just trying to make me feel good.

"Have you been flying lately?"

"Yes, but not as often as I'd like."

"Where do you fly?"

"I rent Cessnas at Boeing Field and fly every few months. I only go when I'm rested and the weather's good. The two haven't coincided very often during residency."

"You're amazing—an ER doctor with nerves of steel, a shooter, and a pilot to boot. I'm not nearly as strong."

"You have to be strong to get into the surgery program. It's highly competitive. You're a star, certainly a star in bed." I smiled.

He laughed and got up from the table. "On that note, I think I better start dinner."

"Dad had life insurance that helped pay for school, but I spent some of the money just to keep current flying so I didn't waste the flight training. After I get a real job, I'd like to buy a plane."

Brett pulled two salads out of the small refrigerator and went topside to light a propane grill attached to the aft railing. I stood on the ladder, partway down in the cabin, and watched him from under the protection of a plastic rain fly cut in vertical strips. The strips flapped in the breeze but kept most of the rain out. The smell of the sea, grilling salmon, and the scream of an interested seagull painted my landscape. Warmth from the boat behind me contrasted with the cold rain that found its way to my skin.

"It's easier to grill dockside than out on the water." From my location partway down in the hold, Brett looked tall against the darkening sky. "I hope you like salmon. I bought some deli red potato salad to go with it. How does that sound?"

"They're both favorites."

Our comfortable conversation continued as he watched the salmon cook. After eating a delicious meal, we sat at the table talking. I felt more positive about our relationship. He knew me better, but I was worried I'd blabbed about myself too much. Later, I realized he'd said little about himself and had kept checking his watch.

Brett walked me up to my car with his arm draped over my shoulders. "You smell wonderful. I'll remember that smell, it's intoxicating." I unlocked and opened the car door, wondering why he hadn't invited me to stay. As I turned to get in, he held me gently, a hand on each shoulder, and touched his lips to the top of my head. "Thanks for coming. It was a great afternoon and evening."

Brett stood there as I drove away. When I turned out onto Marine Drive, I saw him still standing near the entrance to Dock C.

Instead of feeling good after a delicious dinner and hours together, I felt like I'd been dismissed so he could get on with what he really wanted to do that evening. Damn him.

Chapter 12 More Complications

The next evening at work, I got a call from my friend Jen Markus. The secretary took a message and told me Jen sounded upset. I hadn't talked to her since my blood exposure. Jen was a neurology resident and a good friend of Lynn's and mine, but we hadn't socialized much over the past year since Jen's wedding. Neither of us liked her husband. He was a good-looking, pushy financial adviser who tried to get his hands on our money.

I called Jen back as soon as I could. Her voice sounded muffled when she answered. She was crying. "Kelly, I need help."

My voice rose with concern. "What's the matter?"

Silence.

"What's wrong? What can I do?"

Jen took a deep breath. "It's Ken, what else? He's always traveling with his brokerage firm or out for business dinners."

"Sorry."

"That's not all. I just did a home pregnancy test. It's positive."

It was my turn to be silent for a moment. "It doesn't sound like this was planned."

"It wasn't. I've been so tired, and this morning I woke up puking. Thought I was getting the flu. Helluva flu."

"It's a parasite. They sure are cute though." I told her about the baby I had delivered and wanted to take home. "She was given up for adoption without even a hug from her mother."

"I'm not upset about the pregnancy so much as a smelly vaginal discharge. I've never had a discharge in my life."

"Bad news. You better get that checked out right away."

"I've been analyzing recent events with Ken. He's gone so much that I feel like I hardly know him. He's always meeting with clients. Now, with this discharge, I'm afraid he's had more than business meetings. I'll kill him if he's given me a sexually transmitted disease."

"That's a disgusting thought. Get in to see an OB."

"You know what it's like to get out of residency clinics even for an appointment. I have a full schedule tomorrow, a conference where I have to present a case, and I'm on call. No time. Would you do me a favor?"

"Sure. What?"

"Could you sneak me into one of those ER exam rooms in the back and do a pelvic on me, get some cultures, and put me on antibiotics that are okay in early pregnancy?"

"I will, but we'll have to be careful. Because of ethical and malpractice issues, Hunter throws fits if we treat each other. It would be best if you sign in as a patient. Then, it's all aboveboard."

"Kelly, I can't do that. It's such an embarrassment. I'd be mortified if anyone found out. I suppose I could shotgun it and order drugs for myself to kill all the STDs, but I don't want to hurt the baby. Besides, I want to know for sure what this is because of the awful implications and decisions I'll need to make if he's screwing around."

"I understand. Medical records aren't private. Anyone seeing your name could pick up the chart and know your most personal secrets. Things are calm right now. Come down quick. Maybe you can get here before it gets busy again."

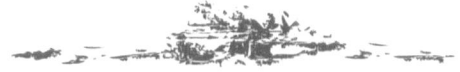

I told the charge nurse I wouldn't be available for a few minutes and took Jen into a private room. She got on the table and into the stirrups. I took a quick look. "The good news is I don't see anything that looks like herpes. The bad news is you have a mucopurulent discharge that could be a variety of infections. We'll do cultures for gonorrhea and Chlamydia and a wet mount for Gardnerella vaginalis and the swimmers."

"Yuck. What do you mean, *swimmers*?"

"Trichomonads. You remember, the tailed creatures that flagellate like sperm in vaginal fluid."

Jen made a face. "Gross. I feel so dirty. How could he do this to me? I'm horrified. I just hope it's nothing that could harm the baby."

"I'm sure they'll do these tests right away. Let's take the swabs to the lab."

Jen and I climbed a back stairwell two flights to the lab. "It's against policy, but I hope the techs will do the cultures without making a record." The tech let me use the stains and a microscope. I got their help to set up cultures and labeled them "test."

The tech said, "Dr. McKay, if you have to get back to the ER, I'll do these stains for you and call you in ER with results in a few minutes. It will take forty-eight hours for the cultures. When do you work again?"

"I'm off tomorrow, and then back for twenty-four the following day."

"Perfect. I work then too. I'll stop by with the test results."

Jen and I both thanked her. I wrote Jen prescriptions to cover all the usual STDs so she could get the drugs started right away.

We walked down the hall, her usual spirited gait and demeanor gone. Jen had many decisions to make. I turned to go back down the stairs and called after her, "I'll telephone you as soon as I get the results."

Jen looked back and hung her head. "Thanks. I'll head out to a twenty-four-hour pharmacy. I don't want to take these to the hospital pharmacy."

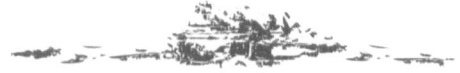

I wanted to call Lynn to tell her of Jen's situation, but the ER traffic prevented my call until it was too late in the night. Lynn had more free time working on Psychiatry than I did in ER. She might be able to give Jen some support. I found

Lynn in a morning group therapy meeting, so she couldn't be interrupted. I asked the clerk to have her call me back in the afternoon.

On my way home, I stopped to buy groceries and passed the REI sports store along the freeway near my apartment, reminding me I had bought nothing for my sister and mother for Christmas.

It was nine by the time I got home. I booted up my computer and Googled REI for easy shopping. I ordered polar fleece sweaters and windbreakers for myself, Kris, and Mom. I knew Kris would like the gifts. Mom might like them but seldom thanked me for anything. She wore her resentment prominently, hating my spending Dad's life insurance money on college and flying.

Kris had come alone to my medical school graduation and honors party. Mom was too busy. Her behavior was irrational, but it saddened me. I tried to never think about it. I didn't need the emotional burden piled on top of the ER training.

Lynn's call awakened me just as I entered REM sleep with a vivid dream of delivering twins in a motel room. "What's up, Kelly? You want me to make flight reservations for Anchorage for you?"

"No. I wish it was something fun like that. I wanted to tell you about Jen."

"What about Jen? Is something wrong?"

I filled her in on the details. "She's pregnant and Ken's been sleeping around. It looks like he gave her a gift that keeps on giving."

"That jerk! I never did like him. A schmoozer. Is she going to keep the pregnancy?"

"We didn't discuss that. I assume so. I got her started on STD drugs safe in pregnancy last night." I yawned. "Just wanted you to know so you could offer some support. I have to get back to sleep. I'm really tired."

"You didn't have Jen sign in as a patient?"

"No. She was afraid someone might see her record."

"I hope Hunter doesn't hear about you treating her without generating a medical record. He went ballistic the last time a resident did that."

"Hunter didn't say anything about a med student suturing my hand."

"That was on the record. They made an incident report of the job-related injury."

"I guess you're right about Jen. I hope Hunter doesn't find out. Jen didn't want a lab record either, so a lab tech did cultures as a professional courtesy. I thought I could do the same. She's one of our best friends."

"I understand all the reasons," Lynn sounded concerned. "I just know what Hunter said. He was ready to throw that first-year resident out of the program over legal liability issues."

"I don't think it's any big deal. I had to do it and would do it again."

"I hear ya. Get to sleep. I'll call her. Thanks for telling me about the mess."

Chapter 13 Another Death

Code blue, ER room 4. Code blue, ER room 4. I rushed to a room awash with people. Someone placed an airway tube, another pumped on the old man's chest. Mona's shrill voice barked orders. "Step back. Everybody clear." She leaned over the body and applied defibrillator paddles to the patient's chest. His body jerked.

Eyes turned to the heart monitor, checking for the return of an acceptable rhythm.

"V-tach." Mona ordered, "Charge to 360. I'll shock him again."

The body, with IVs in both arms and a dangling catheter draining little urine, convulsed again. The monitor showed a flat line. "Damn it! Now he's in asystole," Mona said. "Continue CPR and give him another amp of IV epi."

I picked up his chart to see if I could add information or help with treatment. The front of the chart had *No Code* clearly marked in large letters.

Mona shouted more orders and then said, "Stop resuscitation. Time of death, zero-six hundred."

The team quit after attempting all measures to save him.

Flat line.

Silence.

The room emptied.

A nurse said to me, "Kelly, we never should have coded him. Obvious cancer. He should have been allowed to die in peace without all that violence."

"Who initiated the code?"

"Dr. Maddox. She knew he was on tube feedings and in hospice. I told her he was a no code."

A med student commented in a whisper to the two of us, "Mona told me she didn't want anyone to die under her care. It looks bad."

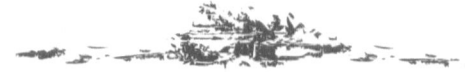

An hour later, Hunter burned Mona for trying to resuscitate a man who had a living will and was near death from cancer. "So, Dr. Maddox, do you realize you could be charged with assault? You provided expensive, invasive medical procedures to a patient who had refused end-of-life resuscitation."

"I walked in on a cardiac arrest and followed protocol." Mona claimed, "I didn't know he was a no code." She glared at the nurse and med student who had talked to me. They knew the truth.

"I have his chart." Dr. Hunter held the chart up for all to see. "You'd have to be blind not to see this order."

Mona shrugged.

"Dr. Maddox, this is the second time you've done this. Even if you begin resuscitation and find the order, you are mandated to stop. We've discussed this numerous times. You are setting a terrible example for med students and others. Stop playing God!"

His steely eyes could have pierced metal. "Have a presentation on legal aspects of end-of-life care ready for the Friday conference." Hunter threw the chart on the desk.

I checked with the lab tech regarding Jen's culture results before going home. Not good. After sleeping ten hours, I called with the news. "You have chlamydia and gonorrhea."

"Gross. That son of a bitch. Am I covered adequately with the meds you gave me?"

"You are. Have you seen Ken?"

"He was out of town until two nights ago. When I got home from the hospital, I was feeling bummed out, and there he sat watching TV with a drink in his hand. He was friendly, as though nothing was wrong."

"Bastard."

"I slapped the drink out of his stinking hand and told him I was pregnant and infected. I said if he had given me hepatitis or worse, I'd see him dead."

I listened in silence.

Jen raved on and on. "He's been living off me and screwing other women. How could he expose me and the baby to disease like that?" The pitch of her voice rising, she said, "He grabbed my arms and squeezed them so tight I've big bruises. Said it was my fault I was pregnant, and he hoped I'd abort so he wouldn't have to deal with a kid."

"You saw his true colors."

"I told him to get out." Jen took a big breath. "I skipped a morning conference today and got an ultrasound. When I came home at noon after the test, I found him humping some bimbo in my bed!"

"Despicable. I can't even imagine what you're going through. I'm here if you need company or just need to talk."

"It helps to talk. I would have blown him away without a second thought if I had one of your guns."

"It's good you didn't have a gun, or he'd be dead and you'd be having a baby in prison."

"Not if I had an all-woman jury."

"Have you found a lawyer?"

"I have an appointment to see J. J. Barber. She's a prominent divorce lawyer and will make sure Ken never sees this baby."

"He'll ask for alimony from his rich doctor wife."

"I'm sure you're right. It's all about money with him."

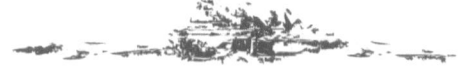

Brett rotated to the VA hospital, and Howie remained at Harbor ER for another month. I felt deserted because I wasn't seeing Brett even in passing, but with Howie's bright attitude and efficient approach, shifts went fast. During a lull, Howie confided, "Brett hates the VA. I talked to him at a mandatory Surgery Department meeting here today. He said he is quitting the program."

"Irrational."

"That's what I told him."

Our conversation about Brett ended when a trauma arrived. Later, I called the VA and paged Brett. I wasn't sure what I'd say, but I decided to invite him to go to the shooting range. Maybe I could distract and cheer him. How could he quit after all the years and effort he's put in?

"Warren here." From the tone of his voice, I thought he might add, "What do you want?" Instead, his voice softened. "Hi, Kel. Good to hear your voice. Sorry I didn't call you. What's up?"

"I'm going shooting this weekend. Do you want to join me for target practice?"

"Sure. Saturday afternoon after a little sleep would work for me. I wouldn't want to be around a tired woman with a gun in her hand."

"Call me when you wake up. There's a shooting range in Kenmore, not far from my apartment."

Not a very friendly or satisfying conversation, but at least I'd get to see him again. Maybe I could convince him not to quit.

I went back to my patients and called Duke Bradshaw, the radiology resident, for a CT report. The friendly Montana cowboy gave me the information I needed and told me he'd be working at a large hospital in Great Falls in July, back home with his horses. The happiness in his voice made me wonder why I wanted to stay here when I could go anywhere at the end of residency.

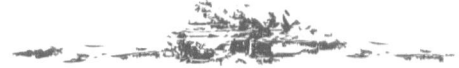

A typical week in the ER ended in tragedy on Friday night with circumstances that made me wonder why I'd ever pick up a gun again. Three people from a wedding party, including the bride, died of gunshot wounds at the hand of her jilted boyfriend.

I thought of their families' sadness after I arrived safely at home and pulled out my two handguns to prepare for target practice. I checked ammo stores before going to sleep, looking forward to seeing Brett in the afternoon.

At 10 p.m., I turned over and looked at the clock. I'd slept all day and into the night.

Brett hadn't called.

I called his cell.

No answer. I left a message.

Was he too tired? Was he down on the sailboat where cell reception is poor? Did he forget?

I got up, fixed a sandwich, and drank some OJ.

At 11 p.m., I finally got in my car and drove past his apartment. No car. He wasn't home.

At Shilshole Bay Marina, I parked and walked to the Dock C gate. The *Chippie* sat silent and dark. No lights on inside. No car in the parking lot.

I drove a few miles to the VA hospital and through the doctors' parking lot. No sign of his car.

I made my way north, meandering on side streets, ruminating about Brett and my stupid stalking behavior. Near Harbor, I turned uphill to take Broadway north to Ravenna, to Eastlake, and then home.

Well-dressed people exited restaurants and walked along the artsy part of Broadway. Farther north, young people in black stood in smoky huddles. I recognized no one. Jamie, the little waif with the ladybug tattoo, came to mind. A horrible situation, with no one to help her.

Chapter 14 More Lies

Commotion and emotion filled the ER when the holidays arrived. The chaos consisted of too many drunks, fights, and overdoses. People partied. Some missed old times and being home for the holidays. I hadn't been home for holiday celebrations in years but didn't want to kill myself like some of the patients.

Among the depressed, a teenage male who had had a fight with his girlfriend decided to end it all. The poor kid took a whole bottle of Sine Off, thinking it sounded like a fatal final statement. He should have read the label. It was for sinus symptoms.

His mother dragged her tremulous son to the ER, berating him. "No girl is worth losing your life over. You should have dumped her before she dumped you."

His heart raced. His mouth was so dry he could barely speak. The boy stared at his mother's blurred face through dilated pupils.

I didn't need to give him a lecture. His mother had done a fine job.

He assured me he no longer wanted to kill himself and would follow up with a counselor.

I discharged him to his mother, who was mad at us for not pumping her son's stomach to teach him a lesson. Her furious words followed him out the door.

During my busy shift, we had car accidents from intoxication, unlucky people injured while trying to break up drunken brawls—a broad mix of problems related to bad judgment and excess mixed with the usual common illnesses. Howie told me he had talked to Brett at a Harbor surgical conference and learned his father was ill. Brett had left the conference to fly home.

After twenty-four hours of non-stop patients, I still had two hours of dictations to complete following Dr. Hunter's morning report. Twenty-four hours off was not enough time to rejuvenate. Many of us overate, snatching high-calorie food from the lounge, on the run between patients.

During holidays, the ER lounge filled with home-baked treats and food gifts of all sorts from friends, other departments, and drug companies; an especially huge basket of fruit and candy arrived from Northwest Organ Procurement. Unfortunately, we worked closely with them, way too often.

Food was the only benefit of working the busiest week of the year between Christmas Eve and New Year's Day.

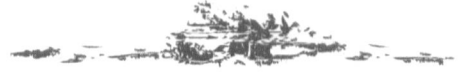

Brett hadn't even called me with a lame excuse for missing our shooting date, nor had he stopped by to say hello even though he had attended a conference just down the hall from ER. Had my insecurity showed so much that I'd pushed him away? I didn't think so, but I doubted he had feelings like those he'd aroused in me. We had had a few dates and good sex, but no real relationship because he wasn't emotionally available.

I worked with Howie a number of shifts and asked his opinion about Brett. "He's smart enough and technically skilled. He's a little shaky in the OR and doesn't defend his decisions well when the bastard attendings pump him."

"He told me he doesn't sleep well."

"None of us get enough sleep, but he makes matters worse by wandering the halls at night." Howie added with a serious tone, "I think his dad might be dying, otherwise there's no way the department head would let him take time off during the holidays."

Had Brett been avoiding me because of his weirdness, or was he distracted by his father's illness? Maybe both. Kelly, the great physician, couldn't figure it out. But, with him out of town, I felt relieved.

I wouldn't be waiting for a call that would never come, and he'd be with his family. Brett wasn't ready for an entanglement, if that's how he felt about our relationship.

I didn't want out. Not yet. If I didn't push him, maybe I could help him through this and we'd have better times in the future.

I set the alarm so I wouldn't sleep all my hours off from work. I crawled out of bed about 6 p.m. and drank a cup of dark French roast coffee with half and half.

The second cup warmed my hands as I sat in my window chair looking out over the lights of the city. The television brought information from the outside world and reminded me of the Christmas Ship Festival on Lake Union. I decided to drive down to the shore and watch. A news flash announced: "The body of an unidentified female was found this afternoon by a couple walking in Ravenna Park. We'll give you an update on the ten o'clock news."

Detective Jones would probably be on that case, too. I decided to call him the next day to see what he'd learned from the other autopsies.

I left in a misty rain for a drive around the city to look at Christmas lights before going to watch the boat parade. Neighborhood holiday lights twinkled. I glimpsed a colorful parade of ships in the distance, slowly moving across Lake Union into the Ship Canal en route to Lake Washington. I drove to the north shore of Lake Union at Gas Works Park and walked down to the water where I could get an unobstructed view of the parade.

Boats of all sizes and types, with lights strung everywhere, moved along the water. Sailboats with their mast shrouds outlined in lights mixed with yachts motoring along with their cabins, bridges, and decks in color. Music and laughter from the boats drifted to shore.

Instead of being warmed and cheered by the sight, I carried a feeling of sadness as a cold wind off the lake swept over me. Why wasn't I on board, warmly dressed, drinking hot buttered rum with Brett and laughing with the merry crowd?

A young couple stood beside me. Their puppy sniffed my leg and said hello with a tail wag. They reprimanded him for being too friendly and commented on the beautiful sight of the boats. I asked if I could hold their dog. The woman said, "Sure, if you don't mind hair on your clothes and licks on your face."

I held him and looked into his darling face. He wiggled, wagged, and let me squeeze him. I needed a hug, but from him I even got a kiss. As I put him on the ground and thanked the couple for sharing him, I looked out at the lake in disbelief. The *Chippie* was motoring past, partially hidden by another larger sailboat, but the lights from the other boat illuminated Brett at the helm. A smaller figure stood beside him, his arm around her. It looked like Mona!

The son of a bitch had lied. He was in town and with another woman. Was it really Mona?

How many other women were open to his charm? How many did he have sex with? Disgusting.

Why did I fall for a liar?

Venereal disease could be fatal. What have I done to myself this time?

Fury drove me to Shilshole, where I checked Dock C. The moorage was empty. Brett's car and Mona's sat side by side in the parking lot.

No wonder he didn't want anyone to know about his personal life; he was dating two ER doctors at the same time. Unforgivable.

Chapter 15 A Sad New Year's Day

New Year's Eve marked the end of twenty-four-hour shifts for residents. That night, triage nurse Shannon wore a little too much makeup. Her flouncy hairdo straggled from a decorative red bow as she whisked patients in shock ahead of complaining patients with minor problems.

Howie admired her too-tight scrubs. When we uncorked our sparkling grape juice at midnight to bring in our sober New Year, he toasted her for keeping things organized.

I agreed.

Fight victims, lacerations, drunks, and patients with medical problems who would rather be home in bed waited for labs and treatments. The staff took the time to make coffee and popcorn.

Duke Bradshaw, a radiology resident from Montana, followed the popcorn scent from his department to ER. His real name is Duncan. He grew up being called Dude, but his doctor friends called him Duke. He answered to almost anything and didn't take offense.

Duke strolled into the department wearing Western boots, a blue scrub shirt, and jeans with a silver belt buckle he earned riding broncs. I pictured the tall, dark-haired, eligible bachelor riding a horse like a movie star.

The ER usually kept Duke busy. He would call CT scan findings to ER or come to discuss reports with physicians and students. We'd been seeing more of him since Betsy, the new California earth-girl social worker had arrived. I noticed she had thrown her Birkenstocks out for a pair of cowboy boots that looked terrific with her long skirts.

The police scanner in the ER buzzed with activity as parties ended and drunks took to the streets. Four ambulances arrived at the same time carrying people from an intersection collision with no significant injuries. They were soon on their way home, except for the drivers. Both drivers went to jail for repeated drunk-driving offenses.

About 2 a.m., a young, assaulted woman arrived by ambulance. Annie, with years on the front line, followed the rushing medics and the stretcher into one of the trauma bays. She stuck her head out of the room. "I need a doctor in here, now. She's barely breathing."

Howie hurried down the hall to the room, hiking his pants up higher, and in his nervousness pushed his dark-framed glasses up on his nose. I loved his nerdy confidence and quirky mannerisms.

Detective Cy Jones arrived with two uniformed Seattle police officers to investigate the assault. "How's she doing, Kelly?"

"Not good since Annie called for more help. She and Howie Hall are in there with her."

"Do you know the story?" Cy stood close enough that I could smell his cologne. He was likeable and calm. A better choice than Brett.

Annie was encouraging me to accept Cy's invitation to the Oregon coast. Annie and Cy go way back, having developed a good working relationship over the years. With Cy, there was none of the antagonism sometimes seen with cops getting in the way in ER. He fit in, a friend and team member.

"The triage nurse told me the patient was dumped in a dark parking lot without ID. People heard her moaning when they were walking to their car. They saw a car driving away but didn't get a description or plate number."

I told Cy I'd check to see if either Annie or Howie could come out and talk with him.

"Let them know we need some information to start looking." Cy called after me, "We'll need good-quality photos to document her visible injuries. A photographer is on the way up."

I met Cy in the hallway after a quick check in the room. "Howie intubated her. She's comatose, with a serious head injury."

"Did they say anything about other injuries? Has she been stabbed?"

"She has a chest wound and a collapsed lung. Blood poured out the chest tube Howie just inserted, so she may go to the OR."

Annie came out carrying tubes of blood for laboratory studies. "She doesn't look like she's been raped, at least no pelvic trauma. I got fingernail scrapings, saliva samples, and skin swabs. Some areas fluoresced, so could be semen. The swabs are in the evidence dryer."

A female police photographer arrived. She followed Cy and Annie into the room. I could hear the low-pitched hum of the dryer when Annie opened the door.

I finished a minor trauma and saw a team whisk the assault patient past, en route to CT.

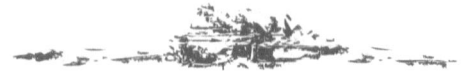

Hours later, Howie barked orders when medics rushed in with an unresponsive knife-fight victim with no blood pressure. The team sprang into action. "Lights! Betadine! Scalpel!" Howie sliced open the man's chest with a swift incision between the ribs below the left nipple. I cranked rib spreaders apart for better visibility, thinking about the last time I'd done that, the night Mona had slashed me.

One stab had entered the man's heart. Another stab went through the ascending aorta, the huge artery that carries blood away from the heart. We clamped vessels, stuck fingers into the holes trying to stop the bleeding, and squeezed the heart, but what little blood remained looked like pink Jell-O water or blood-tinged Ringer's solution. His pupils were fixed and dilated. No blood, no oxygen, no brain function—no save.

Howie took off his gloves and cover gown. "Time of death, New Year's Day, zero-six-thirty-five. A sad New Year for him and his loved ones." He removed his protective coverings, hoisted his pants, and pushed up his glasses. "Thank you for your efforts."

The unhappy day crew surveyed our bloody messes. Most of the rooms were not restocked. Party-animal penitents lined up in the waiting room wanting attention for overindulgence and indiscretions. Alcohol fumes threatened secondary alcohol intoxication of those trying to take care of them. Calls came in to the admissions desk looking for lost loved ones who had failed to come home for New Year's Day celebrations.

Howie went to the adjacent room, where he re-examined Jane Doe and wrote admission orders to ICU. Her brain scan showed swelling. The young woman remained unresponsive. When they wheeled her past me, I saw a ladybug tattoo on her exposed skinny ankle. I grabbed the gurney and stopped them to look at her face. I gasped.

"Kelly, do you know her?" Annie asked, and she looked at the girl's distorted features and bruised neck.

"Annie, we all know her. It's Jamie. The poor little bird Shannon and I took care of a few weeks ago. We got her a place at a safe house."

"It wasn't safe."

Chapter 16 A Deadly New Year's Day

Hand in hand, Howie and Shannon stopped to talk on their way out. He eyed my stack of charts. "You look like you have about an hour of dictation left, Kelly. So sorry. I just finished mine. We're ready to have some real champagne and a special breakfast. Hope you can leave soon. Happy New Year."

Shannon gave me a hug. "Hope your New Year is great. Ours is starting out wonderful."

When Duke stopped by with a box of Montana huckleberry candy and huge bag of pistachios, I took a share and devoured them. Duke raised his plastic cup and clinked mine. "Here's to a Happy New Year. Remember, you're invited to visit Montana whenever you can. It's an open invitation."

After he left, I sipped grape juice and dictated as fast as I could speak. Halfway to my car, I remembered Jamie, beaten and near death. I turned around and re-entered the ER en route to ICU. An ER nurse exclaimed, "Look! Kelly's back already. She wants to work New Year's Day, too."

I rolled my eyes. "Wrong. Not after last night. I'm going to run up to ICU and check on one of our patients." I disappeared through the double doors.

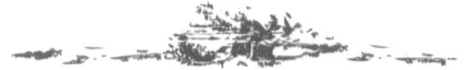

ICU nurses bustled in a circle of cubicles with sleeping or comatose patients. The nurses checked intravenous lines, blood pumps, chest suctions, urinary catheters, ventilators, and hemodynamic monitors. They tracked fluids in, fluids out, and vital functions.

Three young people in adjacent beds lay breathing on synchronized ventilators. All of them were on autopilot, one of them Jamie. Her ventilator cycled—inhale, exhale, inhale, exhale. Her injured brain couldn't even provide the basic function of breathing. The white sheet over Jamie's chest rose slightly, hesitated, and then fell, repeating this over and over. I whispered in her ear, "Hello, Jamie. It's Dr. McKay."

She didn't open her eyes. Nor did she move her fingers when I squeezed her cold, limp hand.

A large tube from her left chest ended in a bubbling suction container hanging from the side of her bed. The fluid looked like pure blood. From a bag above her head, blood ran through a pump into an IV in her neck vein, suctioned out via one tube and replaced via another. Her crewcut had grown out to a stylish short hairdo. A metal bolt protruded from a shaved area on her scalp, connected to one of the monitors. Bruises and swelling distorted her face.

The most recognizable part of her body was the tattoo.

Her nurse adjusted an IV. "Hi, Dr. McKay. We don't see you up here very often. Did you come up to check on Jamie?"

"Yes. I took care of her the last time she was in and liked her. I also felt sorry for her. How is she doing?"

"She just got back from having another head CT. Her brain swelling is worse, so Dr. Carrington put in a bolt for intracranial pressure monitoring. The pressure is high. The chest wound bleeding has slowed some, but I think they're going to have to take her to the OR to open her chest to stop the bleeding and do a skull flap to decompress her brain." She continued, "She must have made quite an impression on the ER staff. Dr. Maddox was also up to visit her."

"Has Jamie's mother been in?"

"No family has been here."

"Where is her mother?"

"We've left messages on her answering machine. The police are trying to locate her."

"I'm sorry we couldn't help Jamie before this happened. Hope she improves."

I walked out, empty inside, a lump in my throat, knowing her chances for survival were slim. I had a lot to be thankful for, but I didn't feel happy on this holiday.

The thought of twelve-hour shifts helped, though.

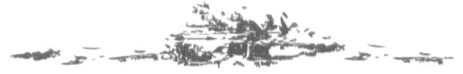

In the darkness created by the foil-covered windows, I stripped off my clothes and dropped them to the floor. A red light flashed on my phone and a green glow from the digital clock played an odd light show on the walls. Red and green, my personal Christmas lights. There were no other holiday decorations in the apartment.

I played the messages. First, a friendly, familiar voice said, "Good morning Doc. It's Cy Jones. If you feel like joining a few of us for a New Year's football afternoon when you wake up, give me a call at home."

Solid, dependable, cheery Cy. Appealing, strong, and predictable. Nice that he called.

My relationship with Brett was so sick, not a comfortable one like I had hoped we might have. When I saw Brett, I turned defensive, afraid I'd say or do something to set him off. I had no time to think. Work wouldn't let me think about anything but work. After seeing the *Chippie* in the ship parade, I wondered if Brett had ever even left town.

The lying jerk.

A second message. "Hi. It's Neville Carrington. Happy New Year. Want to offer my help. Playin' phone tag. You're it."

Now, what in the hell does he want? Why is he calling me?

Before I could get to sleep, the phone rang again, and I wanted to let it ring. "Happy New Year, Kelly." Kris's voice. "Mom and I are sitting here in a snowstorm snacking on lefse. Wish you could join us. When are you coming home?"

I picked up. "I miss you guys and the snow. We had a few flakes here this month. Nice, but it didn't last long."

Mom got on a second phone. The three of us caught up on family events. They always cheered me, except when they begged me to come back to Minnesota. Mother sounded cheery for once.

I told them, "Be sure you get reservations to fly out to Seattle in July. I think I'll have some time off. We can do a little sightseeing around Washington."

"I could hardly wait to talk to you." Kris said, "After a year of dating, Paul finally got up the courage to ask me to marry him. It was an easy answer for me. I want you in the wedding."

"That's great, Kris. Let me know when you decide on a date. He's not a lawyer, is he?"

"No. He owns a snow machine and powerboat dealership."

"I like him already. Bring him with you in July."

"I don't think he can get away then. It's a busy season."

Mother ended by throwing in a little guilt. "I'll continue to write emails even though I don't expect to hear from you."

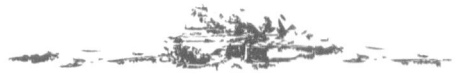

A sharp ring awakened me about 1 p.m. Annie's voice: "Get out of bed and get over here. A bunch of us are at Cy's, and we have a glass of champagne with your name on it!"

Fewer than five hours of sleep left me groggy, but after a little more nagging, I said I'd come. Cy got on the phone and gave me directions. It was just a few blocks away.

A wake-up shower ending with a few minutes of cold water alerted me to the point that I again thought I should have considered psychiatry more seriously, instead of ER medicine. Based on my interactions with a few of the shrinks, most of them needed professional help themselves.

I wondered about my sanity, but it was time to party!

The door at Cy's apartment opened to laughter and cheering from another room where I could hear a TV and a football game. In the small kitchen, two couples were hanging on each other. I recognized the female police photographer. Her eyes sparkled like the champagne in her hand. She gazed into the eyes of a young cop I'd seen in the ER a couple of times. A med student with one of the ER nurses waved with their drinks and kissed, tilting in unison and turning suddenly to see what excitement had brought a cheer from the living room. A dozen people focused on the game.

Cy greeted me, looking terrific in jeans and a green sweatshirt. He handed me a glass of champagne and refilled Annie's, who followed him into the kitchen. I was behind in cheer, but, with so little practice, one glass of bubbly and I'd catch up.

Above the blur of voices and football noise, Cy announced my arrival. Happy and mellow, in full control. His silvered hair, perfect. He delivered snacks and remained attentive to his guests while watching the game.

I waved to Duke and Betsy, who were sitting near the television. I called, "Betsy you look like a real Montana cowgirl in that fancy blouse and blue jeans." They looked happy and entwined. Duke, a football addict, watched every play but paid attention to his girl.

Annie sat down on the floor talking to Nick Ryan, the internal medicine resident who had left his banker wife a month earlier. Everyone's eyes were focused on the TV, including Nick's. Annie motioned to me to join her. I sat down cross-legged and leaned against the couch.

Annie counseled our friend. "Nick, you have to shape up and head home. Make up with her. She didn't do anything wrong. You're the one at fault and on edge." Annie cheered for a touchdown. "Of course, I'd understand if you waited until the game ended."

"I'm listening. I know you're right. Twelve-hour shifts and more sleep will improve my disposition." He accepted more champagne from Cy. "I used to be a nice guy and have fun. Right now, jokes aren't funny, and I don't give a shit about who wins the game or anything else."

Another nurse piped up, "Those are signs of burnout. Doctor, heal thyself."

"She went to visit her folks and will be back in town tomorrow." Nick touched my shoulder and leaned forward so I could hear. "Hope you get the chief resident position."

Annie cut in, the champagne talking. "Kelly, if I were you, I'd go off to some exotic place with sunshine and beaches. Be a *Love Boat* doctor. Don't sit around waiting for Brett." She looked around. "Where is he anyway? He should be partying with us."

I said, "He told Howie he was spending the holiday with his parents."

Good-hearted Annie is a kick at any party but sometimes too quick with words. "That's funny. I saw him driving on the freeway with a girl in his car." She shrugged her shoulders. "I think he's back, or never left."

A sickening wave of doubt swept over me and settled in my stomach. Her statement confirmed my fears.

Annie saw the look on my face and changed the topic. "Lynn told me she's going to Alaska. Why don't you go up there with her? I loved it."

"Lynn makes it sound wonderful. What did you like so much in Alaska?"

I tried to listen to her response through my zigzagging thoughts of Brett.

"It's different, hard to explain. I loved it all, even the long hours of darkness. The sun barely made it above the horizon in Barrow during the winter months. I talked Lynn into going up to Anchorage to check out the job at South Central Regional." The group tuned in to Annie's stories.

"I know Anchorage is really metropolitan Alaska, freeways and running water. Lynn is such a city girl, I'm not sure she is ready for the real Alaska."

"Alaska has an appeal for anyone tired of city life. I told her if she wanted to experience real Alaska, rural Alaska, to try working in Barrow where I lived." Annie finished her champagne. "After I told her the village sewage was picked up by Elephant Pot, a small tanker truck that looked a lot like the water truck that delivered drinking water house to house, she said Anchorage sounded better. I always hoped they wouldn't get the tankers mixed up." The group laughed. "If Lynn's mother visited, she would think she'd arrived on another planet."

We'd all heard stories about Lynn's straight parents. She wasn't with us because she flew to Boston to visit them for two days.

"I remember hoarding stuffed olives at ten bucks a jar, drinking powdered milk, and not eating a salad for months. You couldn't buy lettuce at any price." People seemed more interested in Annie's tales than the game. "I think the winter darkness made some people turn crazy, but I loved every minute of it. People up there are great!"

"No salad?" Betsy's eyes were wide. "I couldn't live without salad."

"If you treat the locals real nice, you might be invited to eat willow tips dipped in seal oil. That's sort of a salad. They tasted good, unique at least, but merely an appetizer." Her gaze drifted to Betsy. "A vegetarian would die on the North Slope."

A television station break interrupted Annie's stories. "Young woman dies at Harbor Medical Center after being beaten and stabbed. Authorities say she was dumped on First Hill yesterday. Police are investigating this death in connection with other deaths earlier in December. All were stabbed. Police are being very closed mouthed about these homicides. It appears there is a serial killer at large who has targeted teenagers in the drug scene. We'll update you as information becomes available."

"Howie Hall and I worked on her." Annie said, "I took care of the last one, too. Are you making any progress on the cases, Cy?"

Cy shook his head. "We have a few leads. None of them promising. I can't say too much until there is a public announcement from the department. That reporter's comment about a serial killer is the last thing we needed broadcast. Now we'll have hysteria and crank calls to sort through, too. It will just complicate the investigation."

The room remained quiet for a few moments.

The game ended.

Jamie had died.

Chapter 17 Mortality and Morbidity

Hunter informed us he'd be doing critiques twice a day, at the end of each twelve-hour shift. I pictured myself doing critiques as part of the chief job and hoped I'd be half as effective as he.

Close to the end of my first short shift, I went in to evaluate a Skid Road bum, an elderly male who'd been "found down." No history. Skid Road is not a desirable address. The term is from the old logging days in Seattle. Back then, logs were skidded downhill to a sawmill on the city's waterfront. The term still held descriptive meaning for homeless drunks on life's downhill road who hung out in the area.

This bearded, shaking, smelly man, incontinent of urine, had small gray critters moving about in his grimy white beard and hair. He wouldn't, or couldn't, speak. Beady eyes looked back at me but didn't focus. I avoided getting too close because of the lice. When I first came to work at Harbor, the nurses had me convinced that lice flew, sort of like small cockroaches. I believed them. I'd never seen a louse or a cockroach before. The staff had fun with young doctors and med students, so I became wary of strange "facts."

This time, I carefully looked in the old man's ears and eyes. He clamped his toothless mouth shut and wouldn't let me look at his throat. Alcohol fumes mixed with other bad smells. Open sores oozed on his legs. We removed his damp clothes and wrapped him in warm blankets.

His temperature at 96 degrees Fahrenheit was low, but his blood pressure was normal. Heart tracing, 100 and regular. A warmed IV of lactated Ringer's solution dripped into one arm. While the tech ran an ECG, I sat down at a desk just down the hall from the patient's room to write admission orders.

The patient's electrocardiogram showed a first-degree heart block, a common benign problem, and no evidence of a serious heart problem. I ordered blood electrolytes, liver functions, a complete blood count, the heart enzyme Troponin, a cath urine for routing analysis, and a sedative drug test. I saw no evidence of injury but added a CT scan of his brain to help evaluate his reduced level of consciousness. Before going on to the next patient, I went back in to check his vital signs. A nurse was inserting a urinary catheter when suddenly his heart rate slowed to thirty.

The crash cart containing all the cardiac drugs sat outside the door. I didn't push the code button on the wall because I thought the slow rate was likely due to a vagal response from the catheter insertion. I wheeled the cart in and asked the nurse to push in a milligram of atropine IV.

Instead of speeding up, he went flat line.

She pushed the code button. An alarm sounded. People came running to help. Mona rushed in and intubated him while we pushed intravenous epinephrine and pumped on his chest. Our efforts to resuscitate him failed.

I left the room feeling uneasy. What had happened to him? He hadn't appeared unstable. What had I missed? Was there something I should have done? I reviewed my evaluation and diagnostic possibilities.

"It was a witnessed cardiac arrest, and we treated him immediately. He didn't respond to anything. I wonder why he died."

Mona shrugged. "Bad luck. He was a despicable creature. Now he's out of his misery. We did what we could."

I evaluated the last few patients with less enthusiasm. The whole staff seemed to be moving more slowly than usual. There were no additional critical medical or trauma cases that came in before the review with Hunter, so I had time to review the dead man's labs and presentation. By the time the patient's labs returned, he was in the morgue in rigor mortis. The labs didn't help, anyway. The tests were basically normal values except for a blood alcohol of 0.08, a mildly elevated white count, and a urinary tract infection.

Nothing that should have killed him.

I knew Hunter would hit me with a death discussion. Worried about the inevitable interrogation, I tried to prepare mentally, reviewing possible causes of death as I treated other patients and dictated their charts.

At critique, my presentation started with an overview of the patient's initial findings. In this case, an intoxicated, confused, elderly homeless person, and, according to Washington State law, legally drunk.

Hunter started in on me. "So, Dr. McKay, why did your patient die?"

"It's difficult to know at this point, Dr. Hunter. With his age and circumstances, it could have been his heart and his years of unhealthy living. He might have had a seizure before arriving here which caused his reduced mental status." I suggested numerous possibilities, including a brain injury and hypothermia.

"Give us a review of the effects of hypothermia." Hunter said, "It's cold and damp outside. In these temperatures, it doesn't take long to become hypothermic."

Hunter was badgering me, but I tried to sound interested and relay information to the med students. "Hypothermia is common in the Seattle area. Your core body temperature drops and body processes slow. Being wet and with even a slight wind, skin cools rapidly." Hunter nodded, listening to my words.

"People die on hikes in the mountains because they aren't prepared with proper rain gear and can't get to shelter. Hypothermia is always a consideration when a patient is brought in after being found down in this weather." I mentioned additional circumstances.

Mona stood next to Dr. Hunter, tapping her foot and looking bored.

Hunter asked more questions.

"It's important to check electrolytes, EKG, look for injury and underlying problems such as low thyroid and adrenal insufficiency."

"Good job, McKay."

Mona turned to Dr. Hunter and rolled her eyes. "Kelly said nothing about the initial treatment being warming. External warming and internal warming with heated IV fluids."

I felt defensive and explained that I had started warmed IV fluids and wrapped him in blankets. "We were waiting for his blood work and his head CT when he arrested."

Hunter said, "This is an unexpected death within twenty-four hours of his arrival here, therefore he's an automatic coroner's case. An autopsy will be performed. The case will be reviewed and referred to the Mortality and Morbidity Committee. That means, Dr. McKay, you'd better be ready to defend yourself."

Hunter turned to his stack of charts and discussed other cases. I didn't listen to anything. Still thinking about the dead man. Asleep on my feet. I had done an adequate job explaining potential factors that might have caused his death, but inside, my gut hurt, like I had just gotten kicked.

I was already dreading the mortality and morbidity interrogation. We called it the big pyre. It's just like the daily critique, only worse, with more inquisitors and a room full of residents, medical students, and registered nurses.

The M & M committee investigated death charts and raked residents from all services over the coals. Pompous asses sat around a table, second-guessing every action. They might as well be lawyers. Maybe these procedures were practice for us for expected future malpractice cases.

Any physician can attend, and questions from the audience are allowed. That adds another layer of stress. Even if you did everything right, by the time they finished with you, you'd feel tortured and wish you'd never gone into medicine.

The last case I presented at M & M was ugly. Mona was there with the rest of them, asking me questions that were difficult to answer. They made me feel worse than I already did over a Jehovah's Witness man who bled to death before my eyes. He refused all blood products that would have saved his life.

Hunter dismissed us, and I realized I hadn't been listening for some time. I had no idea what had been discussed.

I needed sleep.

Mona, at the outer edge of the group, stared at me. I felt her eyes. "Rough shift, Kelly?" She laughed.

I nodded. "Yes. I thought twelve hours would be easy."

"You look terrible. Your hair has that Bozo look I've seen before when you're frazzled. Take your finger out of the light socket and get some sleep so you can be alert and properly pimp the students."

I didn't laugh.

"Too bad you have to defend yourself at the pyre again. Remember, some of the guys on the M & M panel are part of the chief resident selection committee. Not to make it any more stressful of course," she said with a half-smile. "Glad it's you at M & M and not me."

The timing was bad in many ways. I brushed back my hair and needled her in response, "Well, who knows, maybe the exposure will help my chances."

But I knew that when a patient died, the resident got burned at the stake.

Chapter 18 Burned

I read and reread texts and journal articles on sudden death syndromes. There was little more I could do to prepare for the M & M presentation. I had to just suck it up and face the tribunal.

Waiting for a phone call from Brett that never came distracted me from my focus on work.

Dr. Hunter handed me the autopsy findings about a week later, after the morning critique participants dispersed. "Here they are, Kelly. Nothing unexpected, and no explanation why he chose to die at that particular time. Liver changes are consistent with alcoholism. Old lungs, old heart, and a shriveled, alcohol-pickled brain. Nothing that obviously caused his demise."

"Thanks. I'll read it."

"You need to do better than that. Make sure you prepare well for the M & M presentation. You know what they're like." His shoulders slumped. "It's no fun being in the hot seat. I don't want any of my residents to look bad or make the program look bad."

"I understand. I'll be ready." I tried to sound bright and confident as my gut clenched at the thought of being before the tribunal again.

"You're one of the stars. Don't let me down." Hunter walked away.

Mona lingered long enough to hear what he said to me. "You can count on me to be there, Kelly. I might be able to help."

I doubted any help would come from Mona. The day went downhill from there. I couldn't wait to see the end and escape for a few hours.

A frozen chicken pot pie for dinner and relaxing for an hour provided enough refreshment so I could head back to the hospital to prepare for M & M. I hid in the bowels of the library hoping no one would interrupt me. I drank enough Starbuck's coffee to stay wide awake while I reviewed the autopsy and researched abnormal findings in preparation for the interrogation.

Taillights along northbound I-5 clotted into a red line behind an accident, forcing me to take an early exit and make my way home via side streets. I crawled into bed about midnight and got through the following day running on cruise control. A phone call awakened me late in the evening after I'd fallen asleep in my recliner following work.

"You sound groggy, Kelly." It was Lynn Cabot. "Are you up for a little conversation or do you want to go back to sleep?"

"I'm glad you called. I'm really sleepy, but I need to talk to you. The past couple of days have been tough. I love the program and everything I'm learning, but I'm beginning to lose patience with people who come to the ER for hangnails and bunions."

"You're stressed. That happens to me when I don't get enough rest." Lynn sounded like a mother.

"I wish I'd become a park ranger. I could be talking to trees and squirrels."

"You definitely need more sleep when you start talking like that. You need to get away from ER. Psychiatry has been a comfortable change. Sad cases, but not as chaotic."

"Just like in ER, antidepressant and antipsychotic drugs make the world look brighter for them."

Lynn said, "We should dump those drugs in the ER staff coffee pot." She hesitated, "Are you upset over something?"

"Distracted by having to present at M & M. The timing is awful with the selection for the chief position pending."

"Not good. If they haven't already decided, a screw-up at M & M could ruin you."

"I know. With the inquisition out of the way, after this afternoon, my stress level will plummet. Brett hasn't called in a long time, so that's on my mind, too."

"I hope M & M goes well, but you know they can't hurt us now. We're almost done, so don't sweat it. The worst thing that can happen is that Mona will get the job and you'll have to go to Alaska with me."

I felt better after talking to Lynn. She had the ability to put things in perspective.

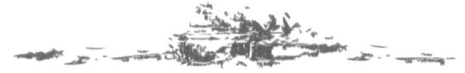

The largest hospital conference room held grand rounds and the mortality and morbidity conferences. My footsteps echoed as I walked the long hallway to the lions' den. A couple dozen physicians and students buzzed with conversation, ready for the conference to begin. I took a conspicuous chair near the front.

By 5 p.m., no empty chairs remained, and a dozen attendees were standing against the back wall. The panel of respected department head experts took their places at the long table on the elevated platform in front, the same table where they had sat for my job interview. Each sat with microphone poised to broadcast all-knowing diatribes and to stab questions at the presenting doctors at the podium to their left.

I clenched my teeth in response to my welling anger. I should not have to go through this again.

Dr. Hunter took a chair beside Surgery Chief Biswell. The Internal Medicine and Cardiology Department heads sat in the center. Neville Carrington, now chairman of Neurosurgery, took the chair closest to the podium, nearest to where I'd present. Even though I didn't like the guy, his smile pulsed me with a calm feeling. I felt a strange, protective vibe from Neville.

I smiled sweetly at each of them, but angry thoughts crowded my mind.

People die.

Sometimes we can't tell the exact cause of death. I sure as hell didn't kill the poor old man.

Two large screens sat blank, waiting for projected PowerPoint slides. I just wanted to get it over with.

The Internal Medicine Department chairman tested his microphone and then announced, "Dr. McKay, you're first on the agenda."

I walked to the podium and displayed my first slide, providing an overview of the patient's age, history, and presenting complaints. Since I'm most comfortable talking to medical students, I smiled and aimed my presentation at them like I did in ER, only this time supplementing what I said with slides. These presentations required a detailed review of the findings and procedures and a discussion of laboratory tests. I described the circumstances of the patient's cardiac arrest and treatment by the code team, including medications and intubation for airway support and oxygen by Dr. Maddox.

In subsequent slides, I showed his laboratory reports. "These blood tests returned about an hour after his death, so they were not available at the time of his arrest. But, the studies provided little help in sorting out what might have happened." I covered my final analysis, including evidence of infection in his urine and a temperature of 96 degrees Fahrenheit.

My last slide showed a picture of the Seattle waterfront in the rain. "He lived beneath the I-5 freeway bridge. Seattle winters are unkind to the homeless. Lights on, please."

I waited for the interrogation.

Dr. Hunter asked, "Dr. McKay, what did the autopsy show?"

"The autopsy did not identify the cause of death. The pathology resident is ready to show slides of liver, lung, heart, and brain pathology, if you're interested in the details, but there was no sign of a life-threatening diagnosis. No myocardial infarction, pulmonary embolus, or stroke. His heart showed slight enlargement."

Dr. Hunter looked at the rest of the panel. They shook their heads. The path resident's face relaxed in relief.

I smiled at him. Now he could relax.

Dr. Biswell asked, "So, Dr. McKay, why did this man die in your care?"

"I believe the most likely scenario is urosepsis contributing to cardiac irritability in a debilitated elderly male. His urine grew out E. coli. He had mild hypothermia and borderline low potassium."

Mona raised her hand in the audience. "Dr. McKay, when I intubated him, I noted his posterior pharynx was gray colored and bled. What did you make of those findings?"

"I didn't get a good look at his throat because he was uncooperative. You didn't mention those findings to me. That sounds like diphtheria!"

I directed my question to the pathologist. "Did you see a gray throat exudate? Could he have had diphtheria? It's the only thing that comes to mind with those findings."

The pathology resident squirmed. He wasn't prepared for the question and scanned his autopsy report. "His pharynx showed hyperemia, no diphtheria-like membrane. I've never seen one personally but would have recognized it. The problem is uncommon these days. I had no reason to do throat cultures. I don't have results to confirm it either way. Sorry."

I asked him. "Is there any way now to confirm whether diphtheria was a factor? I suppose the abrasions on his legs could have been infected with diphtheria as well."

"No. The body has been cremated. Blood cultures grew out no organisms."

"Thanks." I directed my comments to the panel and the audience. "The report from Dr. Maddox complicates an already cloudy picture. In addition to my initial analysis, I will add the question of diphtheria because the minor heart block on his electrocardiogram could have been the result of myocarditis. This problem, combined with other findings already discussed, correlates with cardiac instability and a rhythm death that would give us the indeterminate autopsy findings we have."

Dr. Biswell asked the panel and the audience, "Are there any more questions for Dr. McKay?"

The Internal Medicine chief pulled his microphone toward him. "I have no questions for Dr. McKay, but we need to have a word with Dr. Maddox right after this meeting. Not bringing up this kind of critical information until a time like this is unforgivable." He glared at Mona. "Dr. Maddox, if this was a case of diphtheria, we need to set up surveillance measures. We should have started looking for the disease in others right away."

Hunter's face froze in a frown. "The homeless and immune-suppressed in this community are at high risk. Diphtheria in that group could result in a public health crisis. Others could die."

His face blanched. He leaned toward Biswell and covered the microphone for a comment while glaring at Mona. Hunter added, "It is very unfortunate that specimens were not obtained to confirm this suspicion. Maybe there's a serum titer we could add to the stored blood. If Dr. Maddox had offered her findings to Dr. McKay at the time, we wouldn't have this problem." He pushed his microphone back, a sour expression remaining. "Any more questions for Dr. McKay?"

No one raised a hand.

"Thank you, Dr. McKay, you may step down."

I gathered my notes and looked at the interrogators. Neville Carrington's eyes were fixated on my right breast. He smiled and then, with a questioning look on his face, licked his lips.

Weird man.

The next victim took the podium.

I strode out. I found Mona's face in the audience and added my glare. Any normal cohort would have discussed the findings at the time, but not her. She saved a bombshell for a large audience to besmirch me and the pathology resident. This public barb revealed Mona's serious competition for the chief position and her intent to harm me. I loved that it backfired and burned her instead.

As soon as I reached home, I telephoned Lynn to tell her about how Mona's bombshell had backfired. "I don't know if she really saw a gray exudate or not, but that's what she said."

"Did anyone ask her why she didn't report it at the time?"

"Yeah. The committee ordered her to stay and meet with them. She didn't expect to be in the hot seat."

"Now what?" Lynn asked in disgust.

"More work for the ER. Monitoring yet another problem in the street people, looking for diphtheria. More paperwork. There's no way to look back and document it because the body's been cremated."

Lynn exclaimed, "Mona's a tough one to work with. A month with her last summer and I wanted to poison her before we finished the rotation. She is so competitive, she makes you look laid back."

"Mona's determined to get the chief resident job. I'll have to watch my back."

Chapter 19 Another Fire

Eating microwaved leftover pasta with marinara sauce and sipping a glass of red wine, I looked out over the beautiful Seattle skyline from my recliner thinking about how much I'd miss the view if I moved to Alaska. I lit a candle for ambience and ate slowly, thinking about my options. The prestigious chief job didn't pay much. I couldn't buy an airplane on the wages, but the job would look great on my résumé.

An airplane could wait.

I got up before the alarm and eased into freeway traffic. An oily spray from passing automobiles added to the poor visibility in the morning darkness and mist.

Hunter opened the morning pyre with a smile. Nowadays, even a smile from him made me worry. He raised a hand to quiet everyone. "I have an announcement. You are the first to know that Dr. McKay has been chosen for the ER residency teaching position." His eyes found me. "Take a bow, Kelly. You're the first chief resident in the Harbor ER program!"

A cheer went up.

I wanted to jump up and down but controlled my exuberance. "Thank you, Dr. Hunter. It's an honor."

"Don't thank me, Kelly. You've earned it through your dedication and hard work. All that late-night studying, keeping your cool under stress, and your superb teaching skills made it an easy choice, even though you had fierce competition."

Hunter made eye contact with many in the group, including Mona. "We had excellent candidates to choose from. It would have been an easier decision if we had had two positions to fill. Sorry, Dr. Maddox."

Mona said nothing, but her expression of anger and disbelief said it all.

Hunter's upbeat critique left no one scorched. He congratulated me again when the group was dispersing. "The written confirmation is in your box. In a couple months, we can get together and talk about your responsibilities."

"Great. Thank you."

Getting the job was my last self-imposed bridge to cross. I was ecstatic. I'd made it. Staying with Hunter and teaching would be perfect. But, if I hadn't gotten the job, the way Brett had been acting, leaving him behind would have been easy.

Lynn half-heartedly congratulated me after the critique, then added, "Maybe you're afraid to be out of the university system, out there working in the real world, alone, with no one like Hunter to help. There's comfort in having bright, enthusiastic doctors in training and attendings around everywhere to consult."

"You're right. The system makes it comfortable here. Can I join you in Anchorage in a year or two?"

"The invitation is open. Come any time. The other physicians up there at South Central Regional tell me they like to take time off to kill innocent animals and fish. Frequently, locum tenens slots become available. If they knew when you wanted to come, I bet they'd arrange to have you work while they go off on a hunting trip."

"I hope the teaching job will give me more play time here and opportunities to hike in the Cascades. I could go to the ocean with Cy, but most of all, I want to get back to flying."

"Don't count on it. Hunter's a slave driver."

"It'll be wonderful working with him for another year. He is effective at infusing his impressive knowledge into students. I'll use some of the skills I've learned from him but will apply them with a softer approach. He puts unreasonable pressure on us to learn. That added stress is unnecessary."

"With someone to help him do the reviews, he'll be relieved of some of his immense time commitment. You might change his approach. He may learn from you. Anyway, congratulations. Let's celebrate with a dinner out sometime soon."

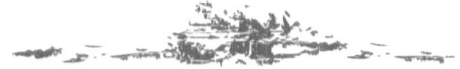

The next day, I felt rested, invigorated, and ready for anything. When I went into the lounge to get a cup of coffee, I found Ben, another resident in need of an attitude adjustment.

"Kelly, how can you look so happy? This place sucks."

"What's up?"

"I try to do a detailed history and be compassionate, but the questions I really want to ask stream through my brain. Like, why are you bringing this child in at two a.m. when he has been sick for four days?" Ben took a breath and spewed more exasperation. "Why are you concerned about your cough now, at four a.m., when you've been coughing for years and smoke three packs of cigarettes a day? You haven't had a bowel movement in six days, but it's an emergency at midnight?"

I listened.

Ben rolled his eyes. "I'm supposed to feel sorry for you? You just drank a twelve-pack of beer and your stomach hurts? You just shot up methamphetamine and your heart is racing? What a surprise."

"We've all been there. Lack of sleep combined with no time to unwind has a way of making everything look negative. Let's take a walk outside for a minute. You might feel better."

He looked quizzical but followed me.

The doors parted and we found ourselves pelted by snowflakes.

"Hey, Kelly, it's actually snowing, snowing in Seattle, awesome!" His beeper buzzed him back to work, but he left smiling after talking with me about skiing.

Small distractions from work can help reduce stress and force us to look into the future. Snow in Seattle raises spirits, like rain in the desert. When I was on a student rotation in Nevada, the whole ER staff ran outside for a few moments just to be pelted by rain.

Mona picked up a chart. "This is the fifth damn drunk I've seen today. I get so tired of them and the teenage druggies. They do it to themselves and expect us to care. Do you mind taking this one?" She handed the chart to me and stomped down the hall.

Years earlier, Mona had voiced bitterness about an abusive alcoholic grandfather. He had lived with her family until he died. That might be why she is so intolerant of alcoholics, but I didn't know why she disliked the drug users. Not being chosen for the chief job probably was contributing to her negative feelings today.

I introduced myself to an ill elderly man who exclaimed, "Only had three beers today, Doc. Been throwing up. Feelin' awful weak."

They all say they've had only three beers.

The gray-haired, unshaven man appeared malnourished. His skin, yellow. No teeth. Exam typical: hard liver, abdomen soft, small amount of blood in the stool. Heart monitor showed a regular rhythm, rate 100. Cirrhosis, failing liver, sad existence.

I finished my exam and started an IV infusion with a "banana bag" of fluid that was colored yellow from the added vitamins. While he rested, I arranged his admission to Internal Medicine and waited for his lab studies.

A monitor alarmed. I scanned the monitor screens at the desk and found his room.

His heart rhythm was a flat line!

I jumped out of my chair and ran to his room hoping to find a chest lead had fallen off, generating the screaming monitor alarm.

Mona rushed into the room and pushed the code alarm on the wall. The automated system summoned help. Others arrived as we slipped a board under his back to make chest compressions more effective. Mona pumped on his chest while I took the intubation equipment and slid a tube into his airway. After her performance at M & M, I wasn't about to let her place a tube in any of my patients.

I ordered, "Give him an amp of epinephrine." A nurse pushed the drug into his intravenous line. Chest compressions circulated the drugs.

Despite 100 percent oxygen, effective chest compressions, and the stimulant drug, his heart rhythm remained flat-lined in asystole.

Mona yelled, "Give him an amp of calcium."

I frowned. "Calcium isn't part of current guidelines." I directed the nurses, "Let's put on the external pacer. Bolus him with saline."

Mona butted in. "Kelly, you have nothing to lose. They don't usually come back from asystole anyway." She ordered, "Nurse, go ahead and give him a gram of calcium gluconate. Continue CPR."

The nurse looked at me for approval since I was the patient's doctor. I raised my eyebrows in a questioning expression and shrugged my shoulders. "Okay."

The nurse injected another epinephrine IV, followed by calcium.

We continued chest compressions for a couple of minutes then stopped to check the monitor. The flat line coarsened to wide complexes, then evolved to regular narrow complexes. I checked his carotid artery. "There's a strong pulse."

The elderly man tried to sit up and pulled his arm away from the nurse checking his blood pressure. She held his arm and recycled the cuff. "Ninety over sixty."

I looked into his face. "How are you doing?"

Confused eyes stared back. "You tell me, doc. What happened?"

Mona lingered near the bed, smiling.

"Thanks for the help, Mona. I'm not sure why he'd arrest like this and respond to intravenous calcium. Maybe he's had a high potassium."

"Could be. Glad I was here to help." Mona walked out.

I wrote an order and directed the nurse, "Please call the lab. I want them to draw another set of electrolytes and cardiac enzymes. Ask if his first labs are ready yet."

I called internal medicine resident Nick Ryan, to admit the patient to ICU and told him about the unusual response to calcium. Nick and his student arrived in ER just as the man arrested again. I worked on the patient for twenty minutes with Mona, Nick, and the med student. We tried calcium again and an external pacer.

He remained flat line.

Mona pulled the sheet up, covering the old man's face. "Kelly, you're going to have to get a better handle on your patients. This is the second patient you've lost recently."

I walked out of the room feeling defensive and angry. I picked up the old man's chart to dictate a death note, then had the lab draw a couple of tubes of blood post mortem to hold for possible additional studies. Maybe Hunter would have some ideas I hadn't considered.

The initial labs showed a bilirubin elevation and liver test abnormalities commonly seen in alcoholics. Nothing to explain the cardiac arrest. There were no findings to suggest something as uncommon as diphtheria. His throat had appeared normal when I put in the endotracheal tube.

I'd have to wait for the autopsy.

Hunter burned me during morning report. I'd tried to prepare myself for his interrogation while caring for other patients. I presented the case to everyone and added, "I'm confused by this patient. His potassium came back normal, yet he responded to calcium after going into asystole. You might see this in a high potassium with muscle trauma or someone in kidney failure, but he had neither."

Hunter said, "True, or with excessive oral or IV dosing. Had you given him potassium in his IV?"

"No." I waited for more thoughts from the master.

Hunter came down hard on me for the unexplained death. "Dr. McKay, it appears you have no idea why this man died." He asked pointed questions about conditions that might be improved with IV calcium, then added, "Give us five possible causes for his death."

Residents and medical students from the last shift, and the new crew starting the day, stood at attention. Listening. Watching me. Waiting. Probably anticipating similar treatment from him in the future.

My brain stalled after speeding through so many patients in the preceding twelve hours. "My immediate thought was that I'd missed a head injury or some other obvious diagnosis. Certainly, he was lethargic, but not obtunded. His airway was not compromised even though he had pneumonia." I paused, looking at Hunter. "I didn't think it was a respiratory death. Maybe aspiration, but when I intubated him, there was no evidence that he had vomited or had any airway abnormality."

Hunter frowned. "What else? You've omitted some serious possibilities."

"Well, something metabolic, a seizure from alcohol withdrawal, low blood sugar, poison such as ingestion of ethylene glycol, antifreeze."

Hunter softened. "Good job, Dr. McKay, that's more than five. How about a few more."

"A primary rhythm death from underlying coronary heart disease."

"That is too common. Give me a zebra." Hunter smiled at the group, seeming to enjoy his interrogation, which made me more uncomfortable.

A med student asked, "A what?"

"One of the jobs of a physician is to consider all the different possibilities that might be making a patient sick, even rare disorders." In a professorial tone, "Just because you hear hoofbeats, that doesn't mean it's a horse."

I knew what he was getting at. His steely stare unnerved me. I racked my brain for more unusual diagnoses that might cause a sudden death. "Three zebra disorders are prolonged Q-T syndrome, hypertrophic cardiomyopathy with a low flow state, and Lyme disease with heart block."

"Good, Dr. McKay." He looked around the group. "I want all of you to realize we can learn something, even from a death from unknown causes. The autopsy will tell us."

Mona said loud enough for everyone to hear, "This is the second patient like this that died in Kelly's care."

Hunter's eyes stabbed her. "Mona, I heard what you said. There is no indication Dr. McKay's treatment is in question. The case will be referred to the next M & M for review."

I stomped out to the parking garage, and Nick Ryan caught up to me. He put his hand on my shoulder, concern in his voice, "How ya doin', Kelly?"

"Not great. I hate it when people have the audacity to die before I figure out what's wrong with them, and Mona infuriates me."

"I hate it when Hunter singles me out. I'm looking forward to being away from Harbor and the Hunter. My next rotation is to University Medical Center."

"It will be quieter and not as intimidating." I looked at the sky. Snow now mixed with light rain. We walked toward the covered parking. Wet blobs sprinkled my face. "I love snow. It reminds me of Minnesota."

"To me, snow only looks good when it's far away. I never did like winter sports." He flipped up his hood. "Growing up in San Diego, I was warm and loved the beach. I'm anxious to get back to California."

I drove home, trying to come up with more causes for sudden death. What did I do wrong? Was there anything I could have done differently?

The old man's sweet smile returned to haunt me.

His death left unanswered questions. My inability to save him started me thinking about my dead father hanging lifeless from his restraints in the airplane. I had screamed, strapped in the passenger seat next to him, my leg broken, smoke filling the cockpit. The helpless feeling resurfaced even though I knew there was nothing I could have done to save my father or the old man.

On the way home, heavy white flakes struck the windshield. The garage door rattled closed, blocking out the fading light. I sat a few moments, then dragged myself out of the car and into the house.

Red and blue emergency lights flashed across Lake Union along the Aurora Avenue Bridge, interrupting my serene view of the city. Freeway traffic moved in steady lines toward downtown. I fixed myself breakfast and took it outside to the back doorstep, where flakes fell on my face and arms in icy stabs. Sipping rich hot chocolate spiked with brandy made me think of skiing. I ate leftover pizza, enjoying the rarity of snow in Seattle.

White sparkles settled on the red berries and shiny green prickly leaves of a holly tree by my door. Sleep wouldn't come easily after another death and another sentence to appear before the tribunal. The brandy finally slowed my whirling thoughts enough so I could sleep.

Chapter 20 Roasted

After a week of night shifts, I got off in the morning and went directly to the M & M conference room. I hated presenting after being up all night. I stood in back and noted many empty seats, but the committee members appeared wide awake and sat with microphones ready for the attack. After reviewing two other cases, the chairman announced, "Dr. McKay, you're next."

I walked to the familiar podium to face the firing squad. Neville Carrington again sat adjacent to me. He smiled and covered his microphone. "Mornin', Kelly. Sorry you have to do this again."

It was nice to see a friendly face, maybe a little too friendly at times, but this morning I needed him on my side.

"Please begin." The chairman's voice brought me out of my self-deprecating thoughts and back to M & M.

"Good morning. I've had a few cups of coffee to get me started after being up all night working in the ER. I'll try to stay alert and duck your sharpshooting."

The crowd laughed.

It wasn't a joke. I meant it, and they knew it.

"Today, I'm presenting a case from the ER. In fact, another older male, a homeless alcoholic much like the case M & M reviewed last month. This man made his way to Harbor by ambulance. My plan is to present the case specifics and then summarize."

The lights dimmed for slides. My rapid introduction detailed our findings, treatment, and outcome. I asked for questions. There were none.

"I made a slide of the continuous rhythm strip to show you the configuration of electrical complexes preceding his cardiac arrest." With a pointer, I walked them through the rhythms. "Here, in the beginning, a regular normal cardiac rhythm. It changed abruptly to wide, slow complexes that tripped the alarm, and then asystole." I turned off the slides. "I initiated treatment under advanced cardiac life support guidelines. CPR. Epinephrine. Intubation. Dr. Maddox suggested using calcium."

I turned to the next slide and pointed to the abrupt change in rhythm after the intravenous calcium. "Here, wide complexes normalized. They became narrow and faster. A pulse and blood pressure returned. I was surprised at the response."

A voice from a medical student in the front row, "Calcium isn't on ACLS guidelines for asystole, right?"

"You're right. As many of you know, calcium is the drug of choice for immediate treatment if someone has a very high potassium level. Because this man's potassium level done on arrival to ER was normal, improvement with calcium, even if it was short-lived, is confusing. At the time of his arrest, laboratory studies had not yet returned, so we had no electrolyte information."

Mona's voice from the dark room. "You know, Dr. McKay, most alcoholics have high magnesiums. We know that can cause heart rhythm problems."

Lights came on. I saw a few closed eyes, but most heads turned to find the voice. Mona sat in the front row. I directed my statement to her. "Dr. Maddox, you're wrong. Alcoholics usually have low magnesium levels."

Her face turned crimson. "I misspoke. I meant to say low. I guess, like you, I'm not awake this morning."

"His IV bag contained vitamins and magnesium. A low magnesium is an unlikely cause of his death. Besides, his lab returned low normal." I looked around the filled room.

Mona sat up straight, listening as I started my discussion of all the potential reasons for asystolic cardiac arrest plus treatment and mortality statistics. Then, it was as if someone had turned her on. She interrupted me, asking numerous inane questions. "What about Romano-Ward syndrome? Maybe you should explain that." She was doing her best to stump me and make me look bad.

I concentrated on my presentation, but she made it difficult, and she'd stumped me with Romano-Ward. I couldn't recall the syndrome, so I ignored her. I thought she was trying to get back at me for making her sound dumb. Her chair creaked. She appeared agitated, rattling papers and digging in a large leather bag.

Dr. Hunter stared at Mona.

The cardiologist interjected, "Dr. Maddox is talking about a rare disorder of long Q-T syndrome. They do well until their electrolytes become abnormal. Death is usually caused by ventricular fibrillation. They die young. This man was old. Dr. McKay, was he having any premature ventricular beats?"

Dr. Maddox piped up, "I saw some PVCs. I mentioned it to Dr. McKay and she thought nothing of it."

That bitch!

She's lying. I glared at her. "Dr. Maddox, I appreciated your help. I don't recall you mentioning PVCs. I didn't see any. I have a compressed computerized copy of the entire monitored time printed and will certainly look at it. In fact, I can check that right now."

I opened the folder and pulled out tabbed pages. "Dr. Maddox, you must be thinking of another patient. These printouts show no PVCs, only the abrupt deterioration I showed everyone a few minutes ago."

The cardiologist asked, "Dr. McKay, did you order potassium to be put into the intravenous fluid you had running?"

"No."

I fielded more questions from the committee related to possible potassium errors.

They seemed satisfied with my responses. Then, Mona's ugly head popped up again.

I heard Dr. Hunter groan.

"What about hypothermia? You said he was cold. Did you warm him? A patient with hypothermia isn't dead until he's warm and dead." Mona sat back in her chair.

I looked at the vital sign record. "Hypothermia was not present. His temperature was 96 degrees Fahrenheit. That would not be an explanation, but for those of you unfamiliar with hypothermic effects on the heart, I'll review typical findings." I put a normal ECG tracing on the screen and compared it with one showing a distortion of the down stroke of the S wave in the QRS, called the Osborne wave." I pointed to these areas and turned off the slide. "Slowing and other abnormal rhythms may occur. During warming, ventricular fibrillation is common. He showed none of these."

Carrington asked, "Was there evidence of anoxia? A few minutes without oxygen and you can see almost any rhythm."

"His saturation was always above ninety percent."

Mona squirmed in her seat.

The chairman asked, "Does anyone else have questions for Dr. McKay?"

Silence.

"Thank you, Dr. McKay. Your discussion was organized and well thought out, but too many unanswered questions regarding cause of death remain. This makes two similar deaths of patients in your care, doesn't it?"

"It does. After an autopsy and careful review of all findings, no cause of death was identified in either one."

The chairman said grimly, "Dr. McKay, you may step down."

I thought my presentation and responses to all the barbs went well before his summary statement that emphasized another unexplained death. When he finished, I felt his fire.

Chapter 21 On Again, Off Again

Howie told me Brett's schedule at the VA hospital kept him busy, but that was no reason not to call and say hello. I decided to call and ask Brett why he didn't show up for our date to go shooting. I wanted to know and then try to forget him if he had no interest in me.

"I slept through it and was ashamed to call." He didn't say he was sorry. Brett didn't know I had checked for his car both at the hospital and at the boat.

Liar.

In our conversation, he didn't mention his father's illness or leaving town during the holidays, but then, without explanation, Brett began calling regularly. His unpredictable behavior made me uneasy. Should I trust him? I decided to tolerate the behavior for a while in order to spend time with him, a bright, handsome surgeon with great potential as a partner. I loved sailing, and the *Chippie* was the perfect getaway.

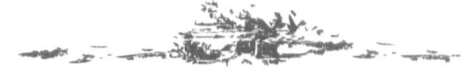

Both ER and internal medicine residents worked on revolving schedules of twelve-hour shifts, seven days and seven nights, and then one day off. Lynn and I ended up on the same rotation after she completed her psychiatry elective. At dinner one evening I told her Brett and I had been spending more time together, often on the boat. "We drink too much and spend hours in bed, not always sleeping."

Lynn's expression changed to disgust. "I don't like him and don't like the way he treats you. He doesn't take you out in public. Ignores you, doesn't call, and then expects you to sleep with him." Her words stung, but I had to admit she was right.

"I feel used sometimes, but until I figure him out, I'll take him any way I can get him." I hated to say it out loud, but I'd resigned myself to his behavior. I craved his closeness too much to give him up.

"I don't like to hear you talk like that. You're making a big mistake. Any solid relationship is based on trust. There's no trust. He's a liar."

I thought about what she said. "I know you're right. I'm more confused now after what happened the last time we went sailing. I didn't tell you about this."

"What?"

"Brisk winds heeled the boat over so far that waves sloshed the mainsail. I told him that he was scaring me and begged him to turn. He laughed and turned tighter, making the angle steeper."

"What did you do? It's not like you could get out and walk home."

"I secured my life jacket, braced myself, and hung on. The angle was so sharp I could barely hang on."

"I'd never go out on the damn boat with him again." Lynn grabbed my arm. "He was in control and enjoyed frightening you, don't you see that?"

I tried to defend him. "Brett looked like he knew what he was doing, but then we hit a large wave from a freighter. The bow dipped into the trough, and I screamed. Brett released the sail and the boat leveled out."

"Dump that son of a bitch. I have no respect for him."

"I shake when I think about it. Now, I wonder why I didn't just dump him after that. But, he turned sweet and friendly, like a wife beater who says he's sorry."

"Get control of yourself, girl. He's a loser."

"I think you're right. He enjoyed the power he had over me."

"Has he ever gotten mad at you?" Lynn frowned.

Her interrogation made me feel like a psych patient in her care. "I have to think. Yeah. He did when we finally went shooting. His hand shook, and I laughed at him. I teased him about it being his surgeon's hand."

"So, what?"

"He slammed a box of shells down on the table like an angry little boy and said he wanted to leave. I thought he was just irritable and tired."

Lynn sat back, disgusted. "With that temper, you need to be careful. Be sensible. You take care of battered women all the time just like I do."

"But Lynn, he didn't direct it at me."

"Kelly, if he's volatile, there is no reason to tolerate that behavior. It's stupid to let him get away with it."

"It's weird. At times, he acts like a guy with road rage. Little things that seem minor to me, like slow traffic or someone turning without signaling, and he pounds the wheel and passes when he shouldn't. But he's never directed his anger at me."

"He may not, but I don't trust him. You don't like Neville Carrington and I don't like Brett Warren. It's a good thing we agree on everything but men. At least we won't be fighting over men."

"In any case, Lynn, I'm happy to be with him again. I'll take one day at a time." I usually felt happy with him. It was difficult to pull away from his charm. "Maybe he needs my friendship."

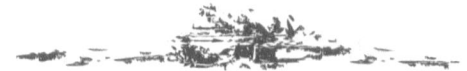

Brett and I went sailing again on a clear day in early February. The wind, laden with a moist sea air, felt colder once we motored out beyond the breakwater. I left him standing at the helm and went below to borrow a knit cap to warm my ears and control my flyaway hair. He smiled when I returned. We stood in the breeze with his arm over my shoulders. I took the helm while he adjusted the sails and set the autopilot. We sat aft in the cool wind.

He unzipped his down jacket, wrapped it around me, and drew me close. His hands searched beneath my sweater, fondling my breasts. Kisses, gentle at first, became passionate, sexual interest growing.

Brett stood to adjust the autopilot, then returned and kissed me gently. He stroked my cheek, my neck scar, my back. His hand felt icy.

I nuzzled against him and pulled up his sweatshirt. His skin was smooth, nipples firm. My hand stroked his bulging pants. We fondled each other while the boat carried us across smooth water, wrapped in his warm jacket beneath a football blanket. The autopilot kept us on course.

Brett occasionally glanced around to be sure we were not in peril or coming close to other vessels. We slipped out of our jeans. I straddled him, trying to hold back, not allowing him to enter. He complied with gentle kisses before his hands on my hips slowly pulled me down onto him. With penetration, orgasm swept us to another realm. I clung to him, breathing fast, feeling him pulse inside. We didn't talk. We didn't have to.

Slowly, we reassembled our clothing, dressed, and huddled beneath the blanket. I pulled up my hood to block the wind. My heart pounded with joy. We headed back to Shilshole Bay Marina.

Brett steered the *Chippie* back to her berth and tied the lines. At a nearby restaurant, we bought espressos that we sipped walking back to the boat. We sat on the aft deck out of the wind, sheltered in the harbor, silent, relaxed, and comfortable, enjoying hot strong coffee as the sun fell low on the horizon.

I studied Brett. Initially, his eyes were closed. He appeared peaceful. I tried to talk about things he enjoyed—music, sailing, food—but he had little to say. He became fidgety and appeared pale beneath a dock light that flickered and came on as the sun set. His hands trembled as he clenched and unclenched his fists.

"Brett, what's wrong? Are you sick? I'm cold and you're sweating."

Angry eyes looked at me. "There is nothing wrong with me. What's wrong with you?" he snapped.

"You're pale and shaky. Are you alright?"

"I'm tired. It's been a long day. Why don't you just leave?"

Shock from his hurtful words made me wonder what I'd done to trigger this behavior. "Brett, I don't have my car. You picked me up."

He jumped to his feet and pulled his car keys from a jacket pocket.

"Let me borrow your car. I'll drive myself home so you can go to bed. I'll pick you up in the morning."

"I'll drive myself, thank you." He taunted me, "Little miss nurse trying to take care of me. I'll let you know when I need help."

I stepped onto the dock. "Why are you treating me this way? Why did you lie about leaving town at Christmas? I saw you in the boat parade."

"It's none of your fucking business what I do or where I go."

He slammed the cover over the cabin and snapped the padlock. He pushed past, leaving me on the boat, and headed to the dock exit.

Brett's abrupt change frightened me. I said nothing and followed him. He got in the car, slammed his door, and started the motor. I got in and snapped my seatbelt. He sped off, jerking the car around corners, silent during the entire drive.

His expression was one of pent-up rage. I didn't like his aggressive driving but feared that saying anything might make it worse. I got out at my apartment and closed the door.

He sped away.

My legs shook after the dangerous drive and experiencing his anger. It was an ugly ending to what had begun as a marvelous day. I needed to share my confusion and hurt from his inexplicable sudden rage, so I dialed Lynn. "Brett blew up after a wonderful day of sailing and screwing. He's unstable."

"He's a jerk. A spoiled brat from what I hear, and you keep trying to explain away his behavior."

"I'm confused by his angry outbursts, but I'm so drawn to him physically, it's difficult to separate sex from caring from love."

"Tell the dipshit to buzz off. Ask yourself, why is a brilliant, conscientious doctor wasting her time with a creep?"

"I don't know. I'm sure it must be my fault. He used to brighten my dark days." I hung up the phone, feeling worse. What could I have done to make him so angry?

I reviewed the day in my mind. A perfectly lovely day. He had acted like he was having a good time and then switched into an angry child. I had done nothing to deserve his treatment.

Chapter 22 Friendship

In medicine, one cannot let personal issues interfere with focus. Patients' lives are at stake. I wouldn't last long unless I learned to compartmentalize. I had to force Brett from my life, my mind, and my heart.

No wonder marriages and relationships often fail among doctors. In the past, any significant problems I had had were work-related, not personal. Brett was my first real test.

Annie and I worked together the day after Brett's explosion. At a quiet moment between patients, she looked me in the eye. "You aren't your usual cheery self today. What's wrong?"

"Brett turned on me last night for no reason. I did nothing to warrant his wrath."

Annie stopped short and put her hands on her hips. "He's passive aggressive, and egotistical like most surgeons, but that man can turn on the charm. With his looks, it's easy to forget what a badass he can be."

"I won't forget."

"Last year, he threw a stinkin' tantrum and I reported him to the Department of Surgery. Lansing did nothing. Said he was having a bad day and excused his behavior."

"Where was I? I missed all that."

"Brett shaped up for a while, but he's as good at intimidation as Mona and usually gets his way. He and Mona used to spend time together. They made quite a pair."

"No way. Mona? That's hard to believe." How could he like Mona?

"I'm afraid you're another of his toys. I wanted to warn you but figured you were smart enough so see through his phony mojo." Annie scanned the ER hall near us. "Just remember, it's him, not you."

"Thanks." My thoughts turned to the Christmas ship parade with him standing at the helm beside Mona.

Annie said, "I saw Brett in ER a few minutes ago. I thought he might be looking for you."

"He's supposed to be at the VA. Usually a resident doesn't leave a facility during his shift." Seeing him at Harbor made no sense to me.

"The Surgery Department asked him to cover here for a resident with a family emergency. Didn't he tell you he was going to be here?"

"No. He doesn't tell me much of anything." I tried to hide my dismay.

"Don't beat yourself up over him." Annie's tone was stern. "Forget him, girl. He's not worth your time."

I left Annie making admitting arrangements for two elderly men waiting for transport to the medical floors. One of them appeared more alert after warmed intravenous fluids. His CT scan showed no bleed, just brain atrophy from years of drinking too much. The man with pneumonia was snoring.

The triage nurse handed me another chart. "Dr. McKay, the psych floor just called to let us know they only have one bed left. What'll we do if we get a psychotic and they don't have a bed?"

"I suppose we'll have to call in more staff and keep the patient here in the ER. Sometimes we can use sedation and admit to a medicine ward. Hope for the best."

"We only have a few hours to go. Then it's someone else's problem." The nurse walked away.

The old man with pneumonia who'd been asleep the last time I checked on him was now awake. IV fluids and oxygen had perked him up. When I walked by, he yelled, "Hey Doc, do you have a cigarette I could bum off ya?"

"Good to see you're feeling better. Nobody around here smokes. You'll have to wait till you're off oxygen." I pulled a blanket from a warming oven kept in the hallway linen closet and placed it over him. He smiled and closed his eyes. "Thanks."

Mona walked by. "Kelly, are you babying the drunks again?"

"I'm just giving him the usual. Vitamins, fluids, and a bed."

She snarled, "Treat them with warm blankets and they'll keep coming back for more."

Mona strode down the hall. Where did she get the energy? PMS?

Weary, I sat at the desk dictating a stack of charts, feeling good about piling them in the out-basket. Unfortunately, my mood changed when the charge nurse assigned Brett and me to an ambulance case. I didn't want to be near him for any reason after the way he had treated me.

Medics wheeled in a young male with back and head injuries sustained when he fell at a construction site. Annie followed the stretcher into the room. With help, we lifted him to the ER bed. As confused and combative as he was acting, he would have been quite a challenge to control except that nothing moved from the waist down. The long backboard aligned his broken back. A stiff cervical collar protected his neck.

Brett took one look at the patient's paralyzed legs and frowned. The triage nurse rushed in. "There's another trauma at the door. A teenage female from an MVA. Ejected. Critical. Comatose. Dr. Warren, I need you to take care of her right away."

Without a word, Brett followed the nurse out of the room, leaving me with the paralyzed patient. Just as well. I hated being that close to him with the tension between us, especially over a critical patient whose life would never be the same.

Brett and I hadn't spoken since his blowup. I had thought he'd apologize. No luck. When the door closed behind him, my thoughts focused on the problem before me.

The young man hyperventilated and pushed at us. He was aware of his surroundings but uncooperative. I quickly examined him. Medics had inserted a large IV in one arm, taped securely so his flailing wouldn't dislodge it. His lung and belly exam appeared normal, but his legs were flaccid. No movement. Paralyzed from the waist down.

"His pressure is 90." The nurse picked up the phone "Get X-ray in room 3. We need a bunch of stat films, including cervical, thoracic, and lumbar spine." She covered the receiver. "Should I get a CT scan ordered, too?"

"Yes, a trauma scan. He may have internal injuries. We need stat surgery and neurosurgery consultation. Bolus him with a liter of saline." I started for the door. "I'll go see who is on duty and bring warm blankets when I come back. Page me if his condition changes."

Annie came in to help, started another IV line, and called the lab for a blood draw. Working with knowledgeable nurses made my life easy. "I won't be gone long. Get usual labs, type and cross. We need intubation stuff ready."

I gave the surgery and neurosurgery residents my initial findings. They promised to meet me in CT. The ambulance entrance doors opened, remained open a few moments, then closed. I caught a glimpse of an eerie orange evening sky streaked with storm clouds. No one came in. No one went out. I wasn't sure what or who had tripped the automatic opener. A fleeting thought passed through my mind. Maybe a ghost came in. Maybe one left.

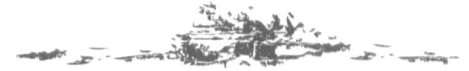

Staff rushed from room to room in turmoil. Someone shrieked and sobbed from the waiting room. The charge nurse whispered in my ear. "Warren's trauma patient just died. That's the girl's mother."

"That's awful. Is anyone with her?"

"Clergy."

I checked the time: less than two hours till the end of shift. Before returning to complete my exam and orders on the unfortunate paralyzed patient, I hurried to the linen closet at the end of the hall. I'd heard from nurses that Neville Carrington liked the dimly lit linen room at the back of the ER for trysts with willing nurses. The thought of hot blankets and hot moments gave me a momentary smile. I ducked inside the small dimly lit room. The door swung shut behind me.

I opened the warmer and picked up a stack of blankets. I heard a noise and looked up into Brett Warren's shocked face. He stood awkwardly on one leg, with the other foot on a knee-high shelf, injecting himself in an ankle vein!

Brett startled. His slender fingers shook, nearly dislodging the needle from the vein before he shoved in the plunger of an unmistakable Tubex syringe of morphine.

Injecting a narcotic mainline!

I dropped the blankets and grabbed his hand, jerking the needle from the vein. "You dumb shit! What the hell are you doing?" My brain raced. "Where did you get that?" Probably left over from the teenager in the car accident that had just died.

Why did a comatose patient need a narcotic? Did he order the drug just so he could use it for himself?

The syringe hit the floor and shattered. He backhanded me and flattened his body against the door, trapping me inside the small room.

Brett loomed taller than I remembered, and an angry hulk I didn't recognize grabbed me. He broke my grip on the door handle and shoved.

I fell against the linen shelves, catching myself but knocking a stack of sheets to the floor.

Brett leaned forward, his face inches from mine. I smelled strong coffee on his breath. His eyes crazed. "This is none of your damn business." His words slurred. "Tell anyone, Kelly, and you'll regret it every day of your short life."

I ducked and side-stepped him, lunging for the door. He flung an arm out, striking me in the chest, and blocked my way.

"Stop it! Help! Let me out!" I shouted. "You can't treat patients when you're drugged on narcotics."

Please, let someone hear me and come to help.

"I trusted you. What have you done?" I screamed. "I hope you're not dumb enough to share needles with anyone. You could have AIDS or hepatitis."

Brett stumbled on the fallen sheets and hyperventilated as he struggled to maintain a grip on my arm. He grabbed my hair, and I couldn't free myself. Trapped. He crushed against me.

I reached the door handle. "Let me out of here, you bastard."

His hands jerked me away from the door again. I flew back against a shelf. Pain blocked my breath.

Brett slurred his words, face contorted. "If I have hepatitis or AIDS, you'll be the first to know, won't you? When your eyes turn yellow and your belly hurts, when you start losing weight, think of me."

"No wonder you're screwing up in surgery—you're a nut case! You can't work and do drugs."

Brett glared and clasped both hands around my throat. "Shut your damn mouth. I'll kill you if you talk." He choked and shook me. Rank sweat dripped down the sides of his face.

I couldn't breathe. I pulled at his hands.

He squeezed tighter.

I'd die if I didn't break free. I had to break his chokehold.

I kneed him in the balls and slammed my hands together, fingers pointed up as if in prayer. In the same rapid movement, I screamed and spread my arms up and out, catching him off guard and splitting his hold.

My foot connected square between his legs.

Brett collapsed to one knee, holding his balls. He tilted sideways enough for me to step past, open the door, and escape.

I raced to the nearest hall phone and paged, "Security, ER, stat to the back hallway," then ran toward the main nursing desk, clutching my neck and gasping for breath.

Two security officers skidded to a halt in front of me, focusing on my neck. I blurted. "Take Dr. Warren to an empty room. He is drugged out and violent."

My voice shook. Tears ran.

Damn it! Stop crying. You're okay.

"Where is he?"

At that instant, Brett bolted past us. I pointed. "Stop him!"

The duo spun to intercept Brett. Each one seized an arm and cranked it behind Brett's back. They locked him into a march step. Brett whipped around, glaring at me. He lunged. In his drugged state, he wasn't much of a threat to the burly officers on either side of him.

The trio disappeared into a lockdown room reserved for violent psychotics.

I asked the secretary to call Dr. Biswell, the surgery program director, to come in and handle the situation.

Shaking so much I could hardly stand up, I remembered Annie stuck with the paralyzed man. Torn between the crisis with Brett and my patient responsibilities, I ran back to the warmer for blankets. Then, on my way back to the patient, I passed the room where officers held Brett. They held him seated in a chair. He jerked back and forth, trying to free himself.

When Brett saw me, he jumped to his feet and sprinted for the door. The guards pulled him back, blocking his progress. "Bitch, you did this. You'll pay."

I sped past, heart thumping, and heard a sharp overhead page, "Dr. McKay, stat to room 3."

Outside the patient's room, I took a deep breath and opened the door. Annie hung up the phone. "Kelly, he's looking worse. Thanks for coming so quick." She pointed at the monitor and vital signs.

Annie's gaze focused on me. She took my shoulders and looked closer. "What's wrong? What happened?"

I bit my lip. Tears welled. Shit, stop crying. I sucked in a breath. "I caught Brett in the linen closet shooting up morphine. He trapped and choked me."

Her mouth fell open. "That son of a bitch. Are you all right? Your neck is red and starting to bruise."

The respiratory therapist helping with the patient's airway management appeared shocked. "So sorry, Dr. McKay."

The trauma victim appeared calm, eyes closed.

"His oxygen is stable, but his blood pressure is lower. What should we do next?"

"I alerted neurosurgery for him. We called Dr. Biswell to come in and handle Brett." I put on gloves to re-examine the patient.

My legs shook. I sat down to calm myself and scanned the monitors while I settled my nerves. "I wish I had recognized his drug problem and helped him."

Annie finished inserting a urinary catheter. She tossed her gloves. "Are you okay to work, or should I find someone to take over?"

"I'll be fine, but Brett's life is over. He'll never do surgery again."

"He doesn't deserve to!" Annie's eyes flashed. "I was suspicious. A damn charmer one minute and vicious as a badger the next." She scribbled a note on her clipboard. "Did it to himself. He knew how to get help. Who was in there shootin' dope, honey?" Annie glared. "It wasn't you."

I got up and studied the X-rays with Annie. "His neck X-ray looks normal on lateral view, but I can't see the lowest cervical level. We'll CT that along with the thoracic and lumbar areas. I see two compression fractures at the junction of the thoracic and lumbar area."

Annie increased the patient's intravenous flow rate. "I gave him a little IV morphine, so he'd be more comfortable." She walked to the head of the bed and adjusted the neck collar.

I finished my exam and talked to the patient about his injuries, explaining my plan for spine CT and a neurosurgery consultation. I explained to Annie and the RT, "His low blood pressure is likely due to the paralysis. Let me know as soon as you get his blood count back from the lab."

Annie dialed pharmacy to deliver the high-dose steroid infusion we prescribe for spinal cord injuries. Even though there isn't a clear benefit, it might help the devastating injury.

In CT, Annie covered herself with a lead apron and remained at the man's side while the scanner spiraled through his brain, spine, chest, and abdomen.

I waited in the darkened control area with Neville Carrington, watching CT slices paint the monitor. "He has a small brain contusion, Kelly. There's no neurosurgical intervention needed there, but I'm anxious to see his lumbar spine." As soon as Neville saw the lumbar area, he phoned OR. "I'm in CT. We have a burst fracture with cord compression from ER. I need to do a lumbar decompression as soon as possible." He nodded. "I'll bring him right up.

Neville whispered in my ear. "I'm so sorry about that bastard hurting you."

Tears stung my eyes. Word travels fast. The darkness of the room hid some of my emotion. I couldn't speak. I nodded.

Annie remained with the patient, ready to help Carrington transport him, while I walked slowly back to the ER, trying to gather my thoughts enough to complete the shift. It took half an hour to finish dictating. I didn't attend the change of shift critique, just signed out to the next doc, and then I walked away feeling devastated, my life forever altered by a lying drug addict.

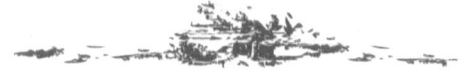

I wept for myself for being so naive, so trusting, so damn dumb. Did the teenager in his care die because of Brett's incapacitation?

I knew I wouldn't sleep. After showering and changing clothes I drove aimlessly and then went to Lynn's. Her car was gone. I drove to Jen's. They were the only two people I would confide in. Our friendships had carried us through many crises. I pressed Jen's doorbell a couple of times, then heard footsteps.

Jen sounded groggy. "Who is it?"

"It's Kelly. I need to talk to you."

Jen threw open the door looking worried and tired, her long hair in tangles. She was dressed in a bright pink jogging outfit with her pregnant belly protruding. She took one look at me and asked, "Kelly, what's the matter? Come in. What's wrong?"

I burst into tears.

She led me to the kitchen and sat me down at the table, where I told her about Brett and what he had done. "He's a goddamned IV drug user, and I've been sleeping with him."

"I don't think he'd share a needle. He's not that stupid. We've all had hepatitis B immunizations, but you could end up infected with all the other STD crap out there, like me."

"I need a hepatitis and HIV screen."

"You aren't pregnant, are you?"

"That's all I need!"

"I'll be tested again before I deliver the baby, but I still think about the possibility of turning positive almost every day. I wish Ken a torturous death."

I looked at my beautiful, sad friend. "How did we get ourselves into such ugly situations?"

Jen tossed her hands in the air. "We're too trusting. Too nice. I'm glad you turned Brett in."

"I had to, but he nearly killed me for threatening to report him." I pulled down the collar of my turtleneck shirt to show her. "I'm surprised I got away."

"And to think I really liked working with him." Jen shook her head.

"I almost lost consciousness before he let go. I'm really afraid of him."

"So, what are you going to do?"

"Maybe I should go to Alaska with Lynn to get away from this mess and far away from Brett."

Jen placed a glass of ice on the table in front of me and poured a double shot of Scotch over the cubes. "You're staying here tonight. Drink this. One shot for you and one shot for me."

"I don't drink Scotch."

"Tonight, you do. That's all I have."

I sipped the nasty liquor. "I wish I could run away."

"That's not like you, Kelly. You'll feel better after some sleep." Jen slathered jam and peanut butter on four slices of bread.

"Here's the gourmet special of the night." She sat across from me.

I took a small bite and another sip of Scotch to wash down the sticky sandwich. "You and I really know how to choose men."

"Yeah, and neither one of us can cook. I hope you like peanut butter."

We both laughed.

Scotch and exhaustion from the long shift, coupled with the emotional stress, soon had me nodding. I finished the sandwich and the liquor and then lay down on her couch.

Jen covered me with a comforter and sat with me until I fell asleep.

Chapter 23 The Morning After

Jen awakened me at six with coffee and a dose of Aleve. I drove home to shower. A glance in the bathroom mirror showed ugly bruises appearing around my neck. When I saw the extent of the bruising, I used my cell phone to take a selfie to document the physical evidence of Brett's attack.

My life had changed. I dreaded facing everyone, especially Dr. Hunter.

En route to work, my sadness turned to anger. Aleve eased my headache, but every time I moved my head, my strained neck muscles reminded me that I could have died at his hands. I hoped my kick to his crotch left him with a reminder of what he'd done to me.

Until the incident of Brett's assault, entering the hospital each day, I'd felt invigorated in the safe comfortable atmosphere, working mostly with likeable people I trusted. Walking into the ER, my feeling of being vulnerable was compounded by the gut-twisting turmoil from the unexplained patient deaths and the repeated interrogations.

My comfortable world had turned dangerous and alien, as if I'd taken a wrong turn and found myself down a rabbit hole. The facility where I had trained for nearly three years was no longer recognizable. No longer safe.

I slipped into scrubs and looked in the locker room mirror. Curly red hair framed my pale, freckled face. I calmed the hair, pulled it back in a barrette, and recalled my grandmother's encouragement from the past. *Kelly, put on a little lipstick and you'll be fine.*

My eyes fixated on my neck. I should have worn a turtleneck under my scrub top to cover the red lines and bruises. I dug into my backpack and found a tube of pale orange lipstick. The color improved my appearance. Gramma was right.

I joined Hunter's report already in progress and stood behind a circle of student physicians, hiding from Hunter. No such luck. He noticed my arrival and announced, "Look what the cat dragged in."

Hunter's dark eyes peered at me over half-glasses. His intolerance of late arrivals had instilled in me the desire to never get his attention by this method. My brain, mush. My mood, terrible.

The Scotch had taken an additional toll. I couldn't have felt worse.

After report, Dr. Hunter asked a resident from the preceding shift to stay and cover for me. His eyes caught mine. Hunter jerked his head toward his office. I followed, not knowing exactly what he wanted to talk to me about. I assumed it was Brett.

Private conferences with Jackson Hunter usually meant bad news. He said almost anything he wanted to say publicly, so a private session often carried grave consequences. Hunter closed the door and motioned for me to take one of the chairs near his desk. I dutifully sat as he rounded his large desk stacked with journals and papers. More of them were scattered across the floor. His leather armchair looked new. I doubted he spent much time sitting.

After a silence of about thirty seconds, which seemed much longer, he asked, "Kelly, do you want to take the shift off and get some sleep?"

I shook my head. "I'll be okay. I need the distraction. You must already know why I'm not having a good day."

"The Department of Surgery filled me in. I'm sorry this happened to you." He leaned forward and looked at my bruises. "Damn him. He really hurt you."

I had to remain angry at Brett and not feel sorry for myself. I blocked my emotions, trying to look strong even though my limbs felt weak.

"It's difficult to turn in a colleague when his whole future is jeopardized by his behavior." Hunter leaned forward. "I congratulate you for doing the right thing."

"What will happen to him?"

"Big things have already happened. Drug use is not tolerated. Shooting up with drugs diverted from patients is as bad as it gets."

I waited for Hunter to continue.

"I was surprised when I heard about this last night. I'd always liked Brett and thought he was doing an adequate job."

"Where is he?"

"Off staff. Out of the program and without a medical license." Hunter looked back at my neck. "Those are significant bruises. Are you going to press charges against him?"

"I don't know." I spoke softly, wondering if this was what it felt like to be in a confessional, though I'd done nothing wrong. "Brett and I were friends, good friends. I had no idea he had a drug problem. He's been on edge lately. I just thought he didn't handle stress well."

"He's in for a lot more stress. He's in deep kimchee." Hunter crumpled a paper and tossed it in a trash can. "His medical staff privileges at all University hospitals have been removed. His contract with the University of Washington Department of Surgery has been terminated for cause. He has been mandated to enter an inpatient chemical dependency program for impaired physicians. In addition, his drug use will be reported to the DEA, and he will no longer be able to prescribe scheduled drugs."

"A lot happened quickly. Will there be a hearing? Do I have to make any statements?"

"There will be a lot of statements. The State Medical Board impaired-physician coordinator will contact you. Hearings are scheduled based on volume, meaning how busy they are. It could be in a few days or weeks."

I stared blankly into the distance. "When I walked in on him yesterday in the linen closet and saw him with the needle in his vein, he said he'd kill me if I turned him in." I fingered the bruises. "I thought he'd be locked up. If he's loose, I'm afraid."

"You *should* be afraid of him. He's free on his own recognizance. I recommend you not only press charges but get a restraining order. It might be enough publicity to keep him away from you."

"He knows I have a gun and am a better shot than he is."

Hunter smiled. "Don't let this destroy you and your common sense. You're a damn good doctor. That brings me to another topic." His expression changed; eyebrows drawn together in a frown. "As you know, any time we have deaths in the ER, the treating resident presents them to the mortality and morbidity conference."

I nodded and gripped the arms of my chair.

"You've had two unexplained deaths in the past few weeks. I reviewed the charts and the autopsy reports." He placed his hand on two charts. "I see nothing I would have done differently, but neither autopsy provided a conclusive reason for death. They were elderly homeless males that died for no apparent reason while in your care."

Hunter listened to my review of the circumstances surrounding the deaths as I tried to defend myself again. I felt my medical career slipping away from me. "I drew extra blood postmortem. We could run additional studies on the stored blood."

"I don't think it will do any good but give it a try. Unfortunately, people die, and we can't always tell why. These two deaths are suspicious. I'm not saying it was your fault, but after a discussion with M & M panel members, we are placing you on monitored status."

His statement flattened me. "Monitoring?" An adrenalin shock rushed through my body. "You think the deaths are my fault?"

"Don't worry. It won't go in your record. We're uneasy about this because you're in the first emergency medicine graduating class. We want no issues on our program survey."

"I did everything right. What more could I have done?"

"Nothing. I've worked with you for two and a half years and trust you. The ER board is forcing me to do this."

"Dr. Hunter, I've done a lot of thinking about those deaths. Neither patient looked unstable, but after missing Brett's drug use, and now with your statement, I'm questioning my judgment. Maybe I missed something."

"Don't be too hard on yourself. People like Brett are very good at hiding things." Dr. Hunter sat without speaking for a few seconds. "Someone once said mistakes are part of the dues one pays for a full life. We all learn from mistakes, especially mistakes of the heart. I'm sorry about Brett."

Be angry. Be strong.

"You need to concentrate on your work. Let's meet weekly to go over everything. We'll do it at the end of each week on Friday mornings, an easy time to remember."

"Believe me, I won't forget. It is a terrible blow to hear all of you think it's necessary to monitor me. Getting the chief resident job was very important. I don't want anything to jeopardize it."

"Please let me know if you need help or if Brett causes you any more trouble."

Hunter got up and shook my hand. He held mine longer than expected and looked like he wanted to give me a hug. His behavior surprised me. In this day and age of sexual harassment charges, hugs were not in the acceptable range of professional behavior. "I want to infuse a little strength into you to get you kick-started this morning. Good luck."

An hour had passed by the time I returned to the ER. The staff searched my face for answers to their many questions. I didn't feel like talking.

While I was in the coffee room with no one else present, internal medicine resident Nick Ryan walked in. "Kelly, you don't look so good."

"I feel like shit." I smiled, trying to hide how bad I felt inside.

"You look more tired than I've seen you before. I heard about Brett Warren. I'm sorry." His eyes lingered on my neck. Nick gave me some much-needed encouragement. Afterward, I pushed on through a never-ending day. Most of my effort focused on maintaining a façade of normalcy. I forced my way through long hours of treating the sick while I was dying inside.

My gut hurt. I wanted to quit. I'd prided myself in not showing emotion after my dad's death and my burns. My ability to suppress feelings had strengthened over years. Working in emergency medicine, I grew strong in the face of turmoil. I studied harder, earned good grades, and regurgitated facts under stress. Now, I smile and encourage patients to take better care of themselves, all the while wishing I had chosen any career but medicine.

In the evening, a nurse and I comforted an elderly woman whose husband lay dying. She held his hand. "We've been together sixty years. He's a good man. He's five years younger. I thought I'd die first." She kissed his hand and touched his cheek. "I'm not ready to face life without him." His stroke extended before our eyes. He stopped breathing and left without telling her goodbye.

She wept.

I didn't cry. I had no emotion left.

Later, medics brought in a twenty-eight-year-old woman they'd resuscitated post cardiac arrest. I talked with her parents as soon as they arrived. "I'm Dr. McKay. I'm sorry to tell you your daughter is critically ill and on a ventilator. She has an unusual type of heart problem, and her heart stopped beating. Paramedics restarted her heart, but she is not doing well."

"Are you sure it's Connie?" her father asked. "She's young and healthy. We saw her yesterday."

Her mother said, "I'm sure you're mistaken. She's too young and vibrant to have heart disease."

I brought them to her bedside. Her mother gasped and threw her arms over her daughter. "Medics did CPR," I explained. "She's been resuscitated but has brain injury due to lack of oxygen during the time her heart stopped. It's too soon to know how well she'll do. We don't know if she'll fully recover."

They stood in shock, clinging to each other, staring at their daughter who was unable to even breathe on her own.

"A drug caused her heart attack. Her friends reported Connie was shooting cocaine when her heart stopped."

Her mother screamed. "She is not an addict! Connie doesn't even drink wine."

I took them to the family room to talk in privacy. "Cocaine causes spasms in arteries. It can cause heart damage, strokes, and kidney failure. People who use it casually don't always understand how dangerous it is, but Connie shows signs of long-term use."

Her parents sat in silence, gripping each other. Her father said, "We didn't know."

The last thing I heard her mother say as I left the room was, "That doctor is too young to know what she's talking about. She's lying. Connie isn't a drug user."

I wrote orders to transfer the young woman to the intensive care unit.

My last patient of the shift was a thin and coughing thirty-year-old male in full-blown AIDS with pneumocystis pneumonia. After admitting him to the infectious disease service and attending a shift change conference, I ran to my car, escaping the flood of sadness.

Chapter 24 A Close Call

At home, the garage door rattled closed. I sat in total darkness, trying to block out stress, disease, and, for a moment, despair.

I dragged myself into the apartment and glanced in the mirror. Would I soon look like the ravaged young man I had just admitted? Gaunt, yellow from hepatitis, with scattered purple Kaposi skin lesions. What awful infection would I die from? What had Brett given me?

The red light on my telephone flashed. Six hang-ups. No messages. Strange. If I had caller ID, I would know who had called. Was it Brett? I didn't want to know.

After a long hot shower, I dressed in sweats. After no food all day, I knew I should eat something. I poured a glass of brandy and spread a stale bagel with cream cheese after trimming off mold. A tiny light on the stove illuminated the apartment. I went into the dark living room to my favorite chair by the window and stared out over the city lights. My brain didn't really register the view. I took stock of my life.

I was on monitored status.

Completing my residency was in jeopardy.

I could lose the chief job before I'd even started.

And, I hadn't even recognized Brett's addiction.

I sat in darkness.

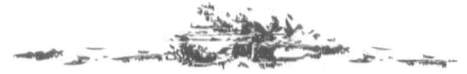

A noise at the door. A key in the lock. Fear swept through me. Instantly paralyzed. I held my breath. Listening. I carefully got to my feet, trying not to make a sound.

I hadn't heard anyone walk up to the door.

How long was I asleep?

It had to be Brett. No one else had a key.

Where's my gun?

I sucked in a shallow breath and rapidly tip-toed into the bedroom. My hand found the cold metal of my 9-millimeter where it lay in a headboard compartment near my pillow.

I clicked the safety off and stood in the doorway of the bedroom. I squinted to see if I'd locked the deadbolt. From where I stood, I couldn't make out the position of the knob.

I always locked it. I had come in through the garage door and hadn't changed it.

A key rattled. Clink. The handle jiggled.

The door shook.

"Who's there?" I called and walked closer to the door, gun poised. Dim light from the kitchen stove confirmed a locked deadbolt. Brett's key fit only the secondary lock, not the deadbolt.

There is a god.

Adrenalin surged. My heart thundered.

Stay angry. Stay strong.

My gun hand swung and pointed at the door. I really wanted to shoot off a round just for effect and to put a little fear into the son of a bitch.

A sharp, abrupt thud shook the door, a kick. The deadbolt held.

"Who the hell do you think it is? I need to talk to you, Kelly." Brett pounded. "Let me in."

"I have nothing to say to you. You nearly killed me. Go away!"

I walked to the door, feeling safe because it had held against his outburst. Through the peephole, his angry face loomed a couple of feet away. His eyes were wild. Spittle sprayed as he demanded I let him in. Suddenly, his body lurched forward, slamming into the door.

I jumped back.

A kick followed.

I yelled, "Come through the door and you're a dead man!"

The casing splintered, and the door swung open. He lurched inside, falling forward, slamming the door against the wall. I fired a round into the floor near the door, raced to the bedroom, and locked myself in. I grabbed the phone on my dresser and dialed 911. "An intruder has broken into my apartment. I need help right away."

"The board shows your address just above Eastlake. Is that correct?'

"Yes. Come through the alley. The entrance is in back."

"Stay on the phone. What's happening now?'

"I'm locked in my bedroom."

The bedroom door rattled. The knob turned.

I screamed. "Brett, get the hell out of here or I'll shoot. The police are coming."

Silence. Heavy breathing, "You bitch. You little bitch."

Retreating footsteps.

"I think he's leaving." I took in a deep breath of relief and listened, my ear against the door.

"Stay where you are."

Within moments, I heard sirens.

I opened the bedroom door with caution and peeked out. I didn't see him, so I sidled along the wall and looked out the door. I saw Brett stumbling down the walkway toward his car.

I listened to the dispatcher, using my shoulder to clamp the receiver to my ear. I fumbled in a pocket for my cell phone. Fingers shaking, I dialed Lynn. She answered on the first ring. The sirens drew closer. "Kelly! Are you okay?"

"I need you. Please come over."

"I'll be there. What's going on?"

"Brett just kicked in my door and scared the hell out of me. I called 911. He's gone. The police are coming up the alley."

Lynn cut the connection.

Two officers I'd met in the ER ran up the walk with weapons drawn. They scanned outside the building and stopped at the splintered doorway." Dr. McKay, is that you?" They walked closer. "Are you all right?"

"Scared, not hurt."

One of them asked, "Was it a psycho from work who followed you home?"

"I wish it was. No, it was Dr. Warren. He just drove away."

"Our other unit cut off a car speeding down the alley. I'm sure they stopped it."

I turned on more lights and kicked splinters scattered on the floor away from the doorway. "Do you want to come inside?"

"Yeah. We'll need a statement. We got a 'shots fired' call. Did he have a weapon?"

"No. I fired my gun into the floor to scare him." I gave them the whole story. Lynn rushed in as we were talking.

They left after completing their report. On his way out, one said, "Strong work! Glad you're all right."

Lynn followed me into the bedroom while I gathered a few things for an overnight at her house. I shoved underwear and a change of clothes in my backpack. "I'd been sitting in that window lounge chair trying to relax and must have fallen asleep. If the deadbolt had been unlocked, I don't know what would have happened."

"Now, what?" Lynn surveyed the damage and turned, eyes angry. "I hope that jackass jerked you to your senses with his violence and lies. They still need help in Anchorage."

"I'm closer to going with you than I was a week ago. Hunter called me into his office this morning, and I thought it was about Brett. That was only part of it. Those assholes on M & M put me on monitored status. They made me feel like I killed those old men."

"That's ridiculous." Lynn clenched her fists. "They chose you for the teaching job, now they do this? I'm going to call Carrington and tell him off."

"How did I not see Brett's drug addiction?"

"We all make mistakes when it comes to love. Remember me and Carrington?"

I nodded. "At least he's benign. I could have HIV and hepatitis from Brett if he used dirty needles or slept with addicts. Today, I had waves of nausea at the thought of turning yellow from liver failure or dying of AIDS."

"Get tested. You need a follow-up blood draw after your laceration exposure in December."

"I'm afraid to do it." I sat on my bed. "I don't want to know."

"Well, that's about the dumbest statement I've ever heard from an educated woman. The bastard better not have infected you or I'll hang him by his balls." She tossed a photo of him from my dresser into the trash. "He betrayed your trust. You aren't pregnant like Jen, are you?"

"No."

"Well, see, you're alive and you're not pregnant. That's something to celebrate! Let's get the hell out of here."

"I envisioned his hands compressing my neck again when he was at the bedroom door. I think I would have blown him away if he hadn't run when he heard the police." Lynn stood in the bedroom doorway while I dressed in jeans and a sweatshirt. "I look forward to testifying against him at the impaired-physician hearing."

"He sure as hell is impaired. I was afraid you'd try to save him." Lynn picked up my backpack. "Let's go."

"I have to call my landlord to get the door fixed and lock changed."

"Let's just close it. Call from my house. We need to celebrate. I have a bottle of brandy and cold pizza waiting for us."

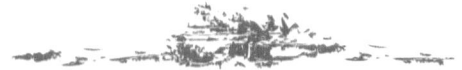

I followed Lynn's flashy Porsche to her apartment. She handed me a pack of Alaska travel brochures to read while she poured brandy and dished up the pizza. "Don't let things get you down. Goodbye and good riddance to Brett." Lynn placed a glass of brandy in front of me. "His behavior changes everything and simplifies your life. Here's to some fun." We clinked glasses.

"I'm so damn mad at the M & M committee members, I can't see straight." I pounded the table. "I'm still shaky from Brett's attack. I'll never trust another man."

"You're not the only dumb chick when it comes to men. I was a fool to date Neville Carrington and have made other stupid decisions in my life." Lynn stopped short and thought for a moment. "Except that Neville really isn't a bad guy. He's a lost soul."

I rolled my eyes. "Oh, dear, what am I hearing?"

Lynn rambled on as we finished our food and drink. I finally said I had to get some sleep.

The alarm awakened us. With her short wash-and-wear blond curly hair, it took her about ten minutes to shower, dress, and be on her way to work in the psych unit. She waved on the way out. "Lock the door when you leave. I'll call you tonight."

I turned and locked the door as soon as she left. I found a note from her stuck to the bathroom mirror. "Kelly, when I had to make difficult choices through the years, I read this little message. Thought it might help you, too." A little yellowed clipping: *If you have made mistakes . . . there is always another chance for you . . . you may have a fresh start any moment you choose, for this thing we call failure is not the falling down, but the staying down. —Mary Pickford.*

I drove to the hospital with a lighter spirit.

Lynn was right.

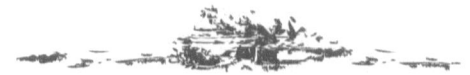

Dr. Hunter squinted at me over the heads of other doctors gathered for his pyre. He called on me a couple of times to explain something to the others, relatively simple problems or concepts. I think he was trying to be supportive and bolster my damaged ego.

After report I walked to my mailbox and found a letter stamped Personal and Confidential. The dreaded letter. I went into the lounge for privacy and ripped open the envelope. Just reading State Medical Board on the letterhead made me uneasy. *Dear Dr. McKay: You are summoned to appear at the impaired-physician hearing in one week regarding Dr. Brett Warren. Your testimony is requested. It is your professional duty to make yourself available to the committee.* The time and details appeared at the bottom of the page.

I sensed someone behind me and startled, still on edge from the preceding night. I whirled to find Mona reading the letter over my shoulder. I snatched it out of her view. "This is none of your business. What are you doing reading my mail?"

"I came here to talk to you. I can't believe you would destroy Brett by turning him in just because he wasn't treating you right. He needed your help, not betrayal."

"You don't know what you are talking about. I saw him with a needle in his vein, shooting up at work when he was supposed to be taking care of patients. Explain that away, will you?" My face burned hot with anger.

At that point, two nurses walked in to get coffee.

Mona left without a word, pushing her way between them.

They looked at me with questioning eyes, too polite to ask what the problem was. One commented, "Mona's been on a roll lately. Hope we didn't interrupt anything."

"Thanks. You came in at the right time. I better get to work. I'd rather take care of a room full of crying babies than deal with Mona." The nurses laughed.

The afternoon hours passed rapidly. High volume and minor problems eased to a halt at 5 p.m. Before end of shift at seven, a forty-year-old male with chest pain collapsed as he entered the ER. He came close to dying several times in spite of our undivided attention. After drugs and two shocks, he stabilized. We moved him to the heart cath lab, where they angioplastied and stented a diseased coronary artery. A life saved. One that would have been lost just a few years ago, before some amazing improvements in technology.

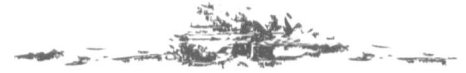

I reached home before eight and called Lynn. She answered on the first ring. "Hello, Kelly."

"How did you know it was me?"

"I just got caller ID."

"Any particular reason you decided to get it?"

"One of the psych patients got my number and address. He's been calling. I liked psych for a while. It was calm compared to ER, with some interesting cases, but this guy has camped out in my neighborhood. How come I'm so lucky?"

"Because you're so cute. The weirdos like you."

"Thanks." Lynn's sarcasm surfaced. "It seems to me you've attracted a few yourself."

"Not lately, except Brett, and he won't be around for a while. I'll be glad when you are back in the ER again."

"Did the landlord get your door fixed?"

"Yes. I feel safe again." I told her about Mona and the summons.

"Think Alaska. I talked to my contact up there today. The guys have a lot of summer plans. There's definitely a job for you."

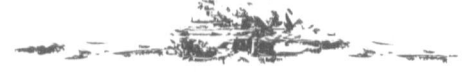

I slept soundly for twelve hours after making sure my doors and windows were locked and my gun resting close by. I was not scheduled until Monday night, one whole day off before starting a week of night shifts, so I walked around the well-traveled three-mile path encircling Green Lake. I carried pepper spray in my pocket but knew Brett was no threat locked up in jail.

After the walk, I called the Seattle Police Department regarding Brett's arrest. I had decided to file assault charges and place a restraining order against him. After accomplishing that and signing some papers, I made myself go to the hospital library to read and check the labs I'd ordered on the last old man who died. He had an elevated potassium. Why, when the first one was normal? I drew it after he died. Most likely, it was high because of the postmortem draw or a processing problem. I researched a few other ideas before avoiding ER on the way out to my car.

At home, I called the Boeing Flight School to schedule a rental of my favorite Cessna 172 for a flight the following day, after a good night's sleep. At times, I still experienced episodes of anxiety at the thought of flying, but once I got in the air, my fears evaporated.

Chapter 25 Fly High

Sunday dawned a typical gray Seattle winter day. A light drizzle dampened the view and my spirits. Flying was not an option with a low cloud ceiling and poor visibility. I brewed coffee. Usually, the smell of Starbucks energized me, but this morning, it took two cups of the dark brew to keep me upright and able to plan my day away from the ER.

The sky lightened midmorning. When the rain stopped, I headed to Green Lake to see if I was up to jogging around it before going flying. I was so out of shape, I ended up walking most of the way while senior citizens passed me. I enjoyed being outside among other people strolling, skating, and jogging. The sound of happy voices was a welcome change from the ER cacophony.

I drove south to Boeing Field at about three o'clock. A few scattered clouds remained. It was excellent flying weather by Seattle standards. The river of traffic on I-5 flowed steadily. En route to Boeing Field, I reviewed flight procedures in my mind. I edged my old Subaru into a tight parking spot dwarfed by large, shiny SUVs.

Inside Boeing Flight School, Ace's strange voice greeted me. He'd been around for years and had seen many pilots come and go. Ace made me smile today as always. "Boeing Tower. This is Boeing Tower. Cleared to land." Listening to the control tower radio made him the most airplane-savvy cockatoo around. His white plumage and crest set him apart from the other flyers, and he often surprised new customers; I'd seen their startled reactions when they spotted him. Even on gloomy days, he seemed cheery.

A wall of windows allowed a full view of planes taking off and landing. In the background, the radio chatter continued. Anyone in the office could hear the conversations between air traffic controllers and pilots. For flyers, sitting by the windows watching airplanes come and go was more entertaining than watching the television that flashed continuous news.

Cessna N5261L sat ready for me. Familiar, like my old car, and a little smaller inside than some of the newer models. This plane, 61 Lima, fit me better, but I still needed a seat cushion to have enough elevation to see over the instrument panel.

I removed a tattered preflight checklist from a seat pocket to guide me through the interior and walkaround check before flying. The last flyer might have forgotten to report a malfunction. I checked everything. With flying, I left nothing to chance or memory.

The engine started on the first try but sputtered before smoothing out. Ground control approved my request to taxi to 13-Left. Near the end of the runway, I stopped and finished the checklist, testing controls in all four extremes: full deflection of the control surfaces, turn the yoke left, pull back, then turn right and forward. Last, I tested engine rpm changes with carburetor-heat and magneto checks, then radioed the tower. "Cessna N5261 Lima ready for takeoff. Request left downwind departure to the north."

After clearance, I taxied to the centerline of the runway and checked the engine instruments one last time as I pushed the throttle forward. The engine noise grew with the increasing rpm's. Faster and faster, then airborne. My heart rate increased with the engine, a feeling of rising excitement mixed with fear. I worked at blocking the panic I'd felt many times. In good weather, the freedom and enjoyment of flying melted anxiety from my brain. Calmness ensued. My level of alertness climbed with the airplane.

I scanned both the area for other air traffic and the instruments before trimming the plane to fly with minimal need for control changes.

Free like a butterfly.

En route to the small Arlington airport about an hour away, I monitored a radio frequency to hear reports, locations, and intentions of other pilots flying in the vicinity. I liked Arlington's friendliness. Its lack of a control tower reduced the distraction of talking with controllers and decreased the fear that big brother FAA would see errors I might make and harass me or jerk my license.

The narrow, paved runway came into view. A parallel grass strip was busy with tow planes taking off and sailplanes landing. In the distance to the east, over the nearby Cascade Mountains, sailplanes rose on slope lift over the mountains. Toward the west, ultralight planes looking like large dragonflies landed on their own grass strip.

My muddled thoughts and long absence from flying showed. I bounced on a few landings but improved as I practiced many takeoffs and landings. After about an hour, I realized the weather had changed. A gust of wind rocked the plane just before landing and forced me to add power and climb instead of land.

The clouds had turned from white to gray. An angry dark layer moved in off the salt water. The sun dipped low on the horizon and slipped from view. Six-one Lima and I departed the Arlington flight pattern. Sunset darkened the cloudy sky as I headed back toward Boeing Field.

I contacted Boeing approach control for sequencing with other aircraft. They gave me radar vectors way out over Puget Sound. I hated flying over water but had to follow their instructions.

The cloud layer lowered as I neared Elliott Bay. Mist hit the windshield and streaked from the prop blast. I located the controls for the instrument lights and turned them on. I also flipped on the landing light, making it easier for other planes to see the small Cessna.

Visibility decreased abruptly when I flew into a sheet of rain. I could no longer see straight ahead. The lights of Boeing Field disappeared from view. Looking down, I glimpsed dark water. A few lights along the shoreline kept me oriented.

Approach control instructed me to contact Boeing tower for landing instructions. My heart raced from the poor visibility and stress of flying out over tidal water. My hand shook as I dialed the radio frequency and called in.

Visibility forward worsened as the rain increased. I scanned the instruments to be sure I'd locked on my assigned altitude. I checked the fuel gauges and engine rpm's.

I had not flown much in bad weather. Dad and I did some "scud running," flying low over the trees to stay out of the clouds. I never felt danger flying with him, only the thrill of carnival rides. He should never have died flying.

My confidence waned. I hated clouds and rain.

I wanted my GPS in case visibility worsened, but I'd left it in my flight bag on the back seat. A lot of good it did me back there. Even if I flew into a cloud, the GPS would get me to the runway.

If clouds obscured my view or visibility worsened, I'd have to declare an emergency. The FAA didn't want non-instrument-rated pilots disoriented in clouds, especially in controlled airspace with all the other airplanes in the area. The tower could vector me down, but it would require explaining to the FAA, even if I kept the plane right side up and didn't crash.

I pulled back on the throttle to decrease power and allow descent along the glide path. I followed their vector and hoped visibility would improve at a lower altitude.

Other pilots talking to the tower distracted my already poor concentration. Even with my noise-canceling headset, the engine noise sounded loud inside the cockpit. The steady rumble decreased as I reduced the rpm's for descent.

Suddenly, the engine coughed. It missed a couple of times and nearly quit.

I lost altitude.

The engine sputtered, stopped, and caught again.

My heart rate surged, and my brain shorted out.

I looked down at the black water.

Rain pounded the fuselage. A sharp gust lifted a wing. I gripped the yoke and righted it, trying to stay on course. I couldn't see ahead,

I'm going to crash. I'm going to die, just like my dad.

I heard his voice. "Kelly, be strong. Focus. Emergency procedure—say it out loud. Say this after me: Above all, fly the airplane. Carb heat. Cycle the fuel. Throttle, full. Mixture, rich. Aux pump, on. Cycle the ignition. Fly the airplane. Select a landing spot."

The only landing spot was in the water, and I couldn't swim.

Even if I survived impact, the frigid water in Puget Sound would kill me.

My mind churned. I voiced his words.

Pull carburetor heat. Damn. I didn't have the carburetor heat out like I should on descent.

The engine was icing in the moist, cold air.

I jerked the knob out, opening a duct for hot engine air to melt the accumulating ice crystals.

Check the fuel, both tanks.

The plane lost more altitude and ran rough, but it didn't quit.

My brain and hands executed the rest of the items on the checklist.

Automated, like doing a cardiac resuscitation. Engine CPR in flight.

The engine sputtered.

I called the tower. "Six-one Lima has engine trouble. Running rough."

Immediate response: "Six-one Lima. Turn left five degrees. Follow straight-in approach. You are three miles from Boeing Field. Cleared to land."

The engine coughed and stumbled. Carburetor heat, on full. Fuel, both tanks. Gas gauges, lots of gas. Throttle, full.

My brain recovered from the instant of paralyzing fear.

If I had to ditch in the water, I had to open the door before impact or I'd never get it open.

Pump the primer a few shots. I had fuel starvation because of carburetor icing. I pulled and then pushed the primer to add more fuel.

The engine surged with each stroke. Now I hoped the engine wouldn't flood and quit from too much gas.

I held my breath.

The engine smoothed.

"Thanks, Dad," I said to the empty cockpit.

My hands steadied, but my knees shook so much I had to take them off the rudder pedals for a few moments. "Boeing tower, sixty-one Lima."

Rapid-fire response. "Boeing tower, go ahead, six-one Lima."

"Boeing tower, sixty-one Lima is running smooth now. What runway do you want me to take?"

"Six-one Lima, your choice. Cleared to land."

I made a slick landing, taxied off the runway, and switched the radio to ground control. "Six-one Lima requests taxi to Boeing Flight School."

I cut the engine at parking and pushed the plane back into its tie down area. Securing the aircraft in the cold, driving rain soaked my turtleneck. It clung to my skin. A chill quaked through my limbs. My hair cranked into tight curls except for the top beneath my baseball cap.

A lineman ran out to help me. "We heard you on the radio. Had us going there for a few minutes. Thought we'd be scooping you out of the water."

I cringed at the thought of my appearance but was glad to see a friendly face, have both feet on the ground, and not be somewhere trying to stay afloat in black, icy water. "It gave me a fright." I looped a rope through the wing ring.

Wet air saturated with aircraft exhaust fumes suffocated me. I felt faint, but the shaking ground and roar of a jet taking off from the long runway rattled me out of my mental fog. I handed the young man the aircraft key.

"Your hands are shaking." He took the rope from me. "Let me finish this for you."

"Okay. Thanks. It was carburetor ice, and it took a while to clear."

He placed the key in his pocket and finished knotting the wing rope.

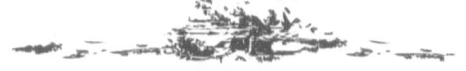

Inside my car, with the doors locked, I relaxed my head against the seat and took a deep breath. Rain battered the windshield, making me realize my good fortune in landing before the storm worsened. I zipped a warm polar fleece sweater over my wet shirt. The defroster cleared the fogging windshield, and warmth from the blasting heater calmed my chill.

I had another chance. I could have died with my job in jeopardy and my career damaged, before being able to fight back and clear my name. I had survived to fight for my job, credentials, and my future, but I chastised myself for forgetting to pull out the carburetor heat on descent. A stupid mistake.

It took a few miles of driving before my knees stopped clattering together. At home, I sipped a glass of brandy and looked down over the rainy city view. I had wasted enough tears. The skies cried for me. My father's strength had brought me through the crisis. It was time for me to display the strength in my genes and get ready to fight the battles ahead.

Chapter 26 Crime Scene

The following day, I had a few daylight hours off before returning to a week of night shifts, and this pushed me out of my apartment to nearby Ravenna Park after a dense, exhausted sleep. Fresh air and sweet scents of early spring blooms accompanied me on a walk along a wide trail snaking beneath tall, moss-covered trees. A shady ravine, covered with a carpet of last fall's leaves and fresh large ferns, moist and green after the passing storm, provided habitat for small scurrying wildlife and chirping birds.

Positive thoughts of taking control of my life solidified as I strolled along, enjoying a change of scenery from the populated path around Green Lake that I usually took. The solitude of Ravenna provided peace and determination to begin my fight.

Enough time had passed that my blood tests for HIV and hepatitis C should be positive if Brett or the slash had infected me. The terrifying thought of a fatal infection ebbed. The future wasn't hopeless. Treatments for HIV and hepatitis C had begun to show promise. Knowing the results, either way, would ease the dark thoughts that crossed my mind many times each day.

If an additional test in a couple of months remained negative, they'd likely remain so, but the unknown would eat at me for a few more weeks. Patients had told me their fear of cancer was worse than having it diagnosed and then finding they were able to deal with it.

Now I understood.

In the past, I hadn't understood why anyone would refuse to have an HIV test, but they would face discrimination and, like me, might lose their jobs. If either test was positive, my life as an emergency physician would be over because of the many invasive procedures that would risk blood contamination to a patient if an injury occurred.

After meandering along a wooded trail and then jogging a distance, I cut through a brushy area, stepped across a creek, and headed back toward the parking lot. Pink rhododendron buds had opened. Stray daffodils on a sunny slope splashed a golden hue near a clutch of dark ferns. I squatted to tighten a shoelace and noticed something purple beneath the ferns, maybe a crocus in bloom.

I walked closer.

As I approached, the smell of death choked the smell of wet earth and flowers. I pushed back the ferns and stared into the face of a dead woman sprawled on her back. A silky purple scarf encircled her neck.

Blowflies darkened the area above her body. Clumps of eggs adhered to her open eyes and mouth, which were becoming alive with maggots. Her white blouse, slashed open, exposed her breasts. A dark fluid trailing fly eggs oozed from a chest stab wound.

I gasped and jumped back, whirling to look around me. Shielding my face from the smell with my jacket sleeve, I scrambled up an embankment and into an open area. I looked back into the creek area, overgrown with brush, and saw no movement.

I felt disoriented and scared as hell. I clutched the pepper spray in my pocket as I ran half a block to my car. Key in hand, I tripped the electronic lock and dived inside to safety. I locked the doors and shook like I had after the flight.

Was the murderer watching?

Had he seen me?

A few people strolled away from their cars toward various trails. Under bright skies and sunshine, unsuspecting people were walking toward the dead woman. Her body lay far enough off the trail that I doubted the walkers would be unfortunate enough to see it. After they'd passed the crime scene area, I dialed 911 and waited.

Soon, two SPD vehicles without lights and sirens parked right next to me. I got out to talk with the officers. An unmarked vehicle pulled into the lot a little too fast. Detective Cy Jones jumped out. "Kelly, I heard you reported this body." He scanned me up and down. "Are you all right?"

I nodded. But I felt weak, and the smell of death clung to my senses.

The four of us walked toward the body as I explained the circumstances. The investigators looped yellow crime scene tape around a large perimeter while Cy walked me back to my car. He said he'd stop by the ER later to talk.

I drove away, hoping my luck would change, and I felt a sense of horror over yet another death.

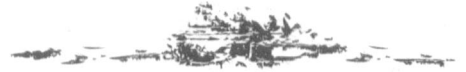

The tech organized her blood-drawing supplies. My arm lay ready for her needle. I held my breath, waiting for that weak, sweaty feeling to sweep over me, dimming my lights and bringing me to the point of passing out. I hated blood draws. I clenched my fist and tapped my foot for distraction.

Her voice interrupted my sensory sweep. "I'm done." She pulled the needle from my arm with a sharp twinge. "You docs tell everybody else to eat right and exercise, but over years of working here, I see you working too hard and stressed."

"I get exercise running around the ER, but it can be stressful." I rolled down my sleeve.

"That isn't the best exercise, Dr. McKay." She smiled. "You'll find the results in a Personal and Confidential envelope in your mailbox within forty-eight hours. Do you want me to add a blood count, chemistry, and lipid panel?" She rotated the blood tubes en route to the centrifuge.

"Sure. Thanks." Having blood drawn triggered bad memories for me related to burn treatment after the plane crash. Thoughts of nurses carrying syringes with long needles. Shots for pain that never worked. A black cloud darkened my vision for an instant when the needle jabbed my skin. What will it take to make me forget?

When I no longer felt the sweaty weakness threatening to engulf me, I changed into scrubs and went to work a few minutes early. My first shift back on nights turned out peaceful, an uncommon occurrence at Harbor ER. Cy Jones came in and talked about the ME findings. "We still have no suspects. Two died at Harbor. Three others off Broadway. All within a few miles of your apartment. Keep your doors locked."

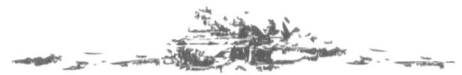

The week of night shifts passed, and I welcomed twenty-four hours off before rotating to working days. Being awake during the day and sleeping at night seemed less exhausting and made it easier to enjoy other activities. Lynn, Jen, and I decided to meet in the late afternoon at my place after sleeping for a while.

I answered their knock. Jen held up an envelope. "What's this? I found it stuck in your door." She handed it to me.

My heart stumbled. The envelope address: *Kel.*

That's what Brett called me during our most intimate times.

Tears welled. I clenched my teeth, ripped open the envelope, and scanned the page. "It's from Brett." By my reaction, they'd already surmised the source.

I handed the letter to Lynn. Jen looked over her shoulder as she read aloud. *Kelly, most of our times together were good times, not just good, very good. I ruined it all. I am terribly sorry I hurt you. Don't be sad. Don't be afraid. Love, Brett*

My throat closed. I couldn't breathe.

Lynn squeezed my shoulder. "The dumb shit should be sorry. He lost the best girl he'll ever meet, lost his position in the surgery program, and lost his license to practice medicine. His sorry ass is gonna be swabbing floors unless he sees the light and goes in for a spin-dry."

"Maybe he's hoping his nice little girlfriend Kelly will support him, buy him drugs, and bail his ass out. He's not much different from Ken." Jen sat down. Her belly bulge pushed out against her long green sweater. "I'm shocked he'd come to your door with that restraining order against him."

"Brett's got to wake up and get dried out." Lynn took my hand. "I hope he remembers you're a damn good shot and his head will be in the cross hairs if he shows up to bother you."

Jen seconded Lynn's statement. "They're all sorry when they get caught. Now let's get this bitch convention on the road." We all laughed, but I felt a dark hand on my heart.

Jen drove us in her black Mercedes with darkened windows. "Let's see if we can keep up with the gray-hairs running around Green Lake." I felt protected from the outside world in the back seat of a Mafia car, at least for the time being.

After a walk, I talked them both into going on a scenic flight with me. Jen sounded excited to go. Lynn never refused a new experience; sometimes she was too carefree, overcompensating now that she was away from her structured childhood and parental expectations.

Our flight took us over the Snoqualmie Pass ski areas and around Lake Washington. Then, we flew north along Puget Sound, returning at dark. We followed the route of my recent flight with engine problems, but this time the air was calm and clear, and the beauty of the area gave them a taste of why I loved to fly.

The sunset glowed orange. The clarifying flight purged me of stress. At the Palisades Restaurant, we ate a superb meal and enjoyed the salt-water view of moored vessels rocking on calm water.

Unfortunately, seeing the sailboats dredged up Brett's image.

Chapter 27 Brett's Hearing

Chairs occupied by miscreant males lined the hallway at the State Medical Board offices. Physicians and physician assistants caught in some dastardly act against themselves, or society sat with their lawyers waiting for a hearing before the Washington State Board of Medical Examiners. Most of their work with impaired caregivers had to do with doctors acting badly. Ethics infractions, mental health problems, inappropriate sexual contact, and controlled-substance, or alcohol abuse topped the list. Easy access to drugs, combined with the stress of practicing medicine, sometimes led to self-treatment and then addiction.

Physicians licensed in the State of Washington received a monthly newsletter detailing Board actions. Problem physicians, their infractions, and the punishment meted out were listed alphabetically. I always checked to see if anyone I knew had gotten the hatchet. Punishment ranged from ordering a physician to write a letter of apology to mandating inpatient drug treatment and loss of a medical license. I never dreamed I'd be called as a witness against anyone, especially Brett.

Brett sat in the lineup. His tousled hair and dark stubble made him look like a common criminal. A heated conversation brought attention to Brett and the short fat man in a brown suit sitting next to him. I cringed, feeling Brett's anger. Along the opposite wall, I felt safe from him as I waited as a witness out of his reach.

The official Washington State Medical Quality Assurance Commission had physicians as members but also included lay people and a physician assistant. Brett quit his tirade and jumped to his feet when a stately gray-haired woman opened the hearing room door and announced, "Dr. Brett Warren."

Brett's attorney herded him toward the door held open by the woman, but not before Brett spotted me. He glared right at me just before they walked single file into the room. Silhouetted by lights within the room, Brett's attorney, with a large pointy nose, led the way. His too-long reddish gray hair flowed over his collar like floppy feathers. He strutted like a banty rooster.

After they passed the coordinator, she requested, "Anyone asked to be present for Dr. Warren's hearing, please enter now."

Just then, Clayton Biswell III, MD, Director of the Surgery Residency, arrived in a rush. He followed me inside to where Brett and his lawyer sat at a large oval table surrounded by Board professionals. Dr. Biswell and I sat out of reach, across from Brett.

The chairperson introduced herself and began the proceedings by reading charges from the report submitted by Dr. Biswell. It delineated what I had told them in my verbal and written reports to the Department of Surgery. In addition, Biswell's report documented legal blood testing identifying the presence of the narcotic in Brett's blood. His report also described Brett's volatile behavior and appearance of intoxication when Biswell arrived in the ER to handle the problem.

Dr. Biswell verbally confirmed the validity of the statement. Brett looked down, his fingers drumming a staccato rhythm on the arms of his chair.

The chairperson introduced me and asked me to describe to the panel what had happened in the linen closet. A sudden barb pierced my heart, but my brain kicked in. Remember, he choked you. Said he'd kill you.

I took a deep breath and hid my hands in my lap so no one would see my clenched fists.

First, I looked straight at Brett. He stared back.

Then, I scanned the faces of the panel members. I told them what I had seen and what Brett had done to me, including the choking episode and his threat to kill me if I told anyone.

I wondered if he could end up doing time due to the pending legal charges, including stealing narcotics and drug diversion from patients to himself.

Brett tapped his fingers on the table and then gripped his chair when the lawyer called a family member as a character witness. Brett's aunt, his mother's sister, spoke of Brett's sad childhood and physical abuse at the hands of his drunken father. There were no further questions or witnesses.

I rose to leave. When I rounded the table near him, Brett whispered, "I'll get you, bitch."

His attorney elbowed him.

So much for love.

I kept walking.

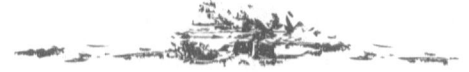

I drove to the hospital and stopped by ER to talk with Dr. Hunter before going home. He was in his office and greeted me with a light tone. "Hi, Kelly, you don't look worse for wear. How did it go?"

"Straightforward. No nonsense. Dr. Biswell and I were the only negative witnesses."

"Did Brett talk with the panel?"

"He let his lawyer and aunt do all the talking. The aunt tried to convince the panel his pathetic childhood and stress from the death of a patient led him to shoot up that day, that he really didn't have a drug habit."

He shook his head. "Some people, you never figure out. Has Brett bothered you?"

"I think you know he kicked in my door and I called the police. He also threatened me at the hearing. I got a restraining order like you suggested."

"He's a sick man. The Board usually hands down its decision within twenty-four hours. They'll expect him to show up for treatment the next day. Then, he'll be off the streets and you'll be safer. I'm surprised he didn't go directly to rehab before the hearing, without waiting for a mandate. It would have looked better on his record."

"It doesn't make sense. He looked awful. I wondered if he'd gotten his hands on more narcotics."

"He'll be in treatment for three months. Maybe by that time he'll come to his senses, but he might still be a threat to you." Hunter shrugged. "It's hard to tell."

I thought we were finished. He didn't stand to see me to the door when I stood to go. He hesitated and had trouble meeting my eyes. "Kelly, sit back down for a minute. I have some unpleasant things I must discuss with you. I don't know how to tell you after all you've been through lately. Maybe that's the reason for the deterioration in your work."

My heart stumbled. I sat down.

"Although the weekly reviews I've done with you revealed no specific problem, I have received almost daily complaints from attendings. The general consensus is they've lost confidence in your care. Even the littlest things are brought up. One of them voiced a concern that your care might be suffering because maybe you too have been using drugs."

"I'll take a drug test right now. I've never used drugs, unless you call coffee a drug. How can they do this to me?" I stood up nearly knocking the chair over. "I haven't changed, but ever since the last M & M, I felt the attitudes of the attendings toward me had changed. They turned cold and critical instead of acting like the teachers I thought they were. What does all this mean?"

Hunter's harsh response stung. "Dr. McKay, maybe the attitude I'm seeing right now is part of the problem. Instead of being a team player, you're becoming a troublemaker. I want you to do some special projects to show me and the others you're determined to improve your care and improve your attitude."

I walked out on him.

That son of a bitch is supposed to be an advocate for his residents. Instead of supporting me, he joined the dogpile.

I drove home in a state of shock, unaware of my surroundings. I even missed the freeway exit and had to backtrack.

Shit. I'm so incompetent I couldn't even find my way home.

Chapter 28 Paranoia

At work the following day, I was too busy to feel sorry for myself. I just did my job. Instead of being energized by working with talented physicians and nurses, I felt paranoid, as though everyone was watching everything I did. Who would report me next?

Had Hunter asked the nurses to critique my care? To call him if anything didn't go well? Does he trust me to teach medical students, or are they privy to my private monitoring too?

The staff saw me meet with him weekly. Why would anyone meet with Hunter? It's usually for problems. An overhead page for help interrupted my negative ruminations. "Asthma in room 2. I need a doctor right away."

I left a stable patient and followed the nurse pushing a young woman in a wheelchair. The hyperventilating, pale, sweaty woman clutched her chest. "I'm Dr. McKay," I said to the woman and helped her get onto the ER bed and into a gown.

"The triage nurse said her O2 sat was only eighty-four percent, so we brought her right back."

"When did you start feeling bad?"

"At four a.m., when I got up to breast feed the baby. It came on fast. I felt all right when I went to bed." I pulled my stethoscope from my pocket. "My son is just a month old and still wants to eat every three or four hours. I was okay at the midnight feeding."

I listened to her lungs and heard no wheezing. "Do you have a history of breathing problems?"

"I have asthma." She took multiple deep breaths between her answers. "I don't need medicine all the time, but we were at a neighbor's last night who had cats." She took a few breaths before continuing. "Cats always make me wheeze. I've used my inhalers, but they're not helping. I tried to wait till my doctor's office opened, but I suddenly got worse, and now I have chest pain." She clutched her chest and started coughing.

The woman spat bloody sputum into a tissue. "The oxygen isn't helping. Please do something."

"Take some deep breaths while I listen to your lungs." She tried but coughed repeatedly. "I don't hear wheezing. Where is your chest pain?"

I instructed a nurse, "Call Respiratory Therapy. Stat albuterol plus Atrovent. Stat chest X-ray."

"It hurts here when I cough." The patient pointed to her left chest "I got the bad pain early this morning.

"Do you have any other health problems?"

"Only being klutzy. I turned my ankle last week going downstairs, so I've been wrapping it."

I removed an elastic wrap and examined her leg. "The ankle is purple, but your whole leg is swollen."

"I know. It's been that way off and on, but worse since the sprain. I had trouble during the pregnancy with swelling." She looked around. "Where's my husband? Can he come in here with me?"

"Sure." I told the nurse, "Please get a stat arterial blood gas and start the breathing treatment. After that, a stat ECG."

"Let's get your X-ray done first, then we'll bring your husband and baby in to be with you. The blood gas is drawn from the artery in your wrist."

"I've had one before. It really hurts. Do you have to do it?"

"I do. I'm worried your breathing problem isn't asthma. It could be from a blood clot to the lung from your swollen leg."

"Are those serious?"

"They are, but there's good treatment using blood thinners."

"No," She gasped. "I'm breastfeeding and they'll hurt the baby. I won't take blood thinners."

"If there's a clot, you'll have to take thinners. It's the only way to treat it and save your life."

"My husband won't let me. He's into natural herbs and healthy living. I know he wouldn't approve." She looked more frightened and clutched her chest. "I had to beg him to bring me here. He wanted to give me camphor tea."

I shook my head, knowing there would be more trouble ahead. "We need to talk more, but based on what I know now, I believe you had a clot in your leg that moved to your lungs."

"Please don't do any tests I don't really need. We don't have good health insurance. I even delivered the baby at home." She smiled, "He's such a proud papa."

A nurse brought in a tall thin man resembling a stick bug dressed in a green jogging suit, carrying a swaddled baby in the crook of one arm. The man looked like a skeletal marathon runner. I explained my concern for his wife and her dangerous condition.

As she predicted, he said he'd allow no treatment that would alter his wife's breast milk. "Make the diagnosis and then we'll decide. No drugs till then."

"Medical standards mandate we start heparin now. It might prevent progression of a clot and possibly stop more pieces from breaking loose and going to the lung."

"Damn the medical standards! I said no." The baby cried out in a piercing tone.

"Blood clots can be fatal," I began to explain, but he cut me off.

"No way, lady," his tone derogatory. He towered over me. "You don't even know if she has a clot. Patients have rights, you know."

I left the room with her breathing on the nebulizer. His ranting and pacing added to her anxiety, mine, and the baby's. I went back in the room, blood gas in hand. "The oxygen is low. She's hyperventilating yet unable to raise the level. I called a pulmonary attending to discuss the case with him. He agrees with my recommendations."

I didn't tell the patient and her husband exactly what the specialist said. He added to my stress by saying, "Dr. McKay, why are you calling me? You know what to do. Give her a loading dose of heparin and do a contrast chest CT scan."

I explained, "They're refusing heparin until we get a diagnosis."

"Do whatever you want. You don't need me. Just call Medicine and let a resident admit her."

I showed the patient and her husband her normal chest X-ray. "She has no pneumonia and no collapsed lung, but clots don't show on X-ray. That's why we have to do the CT scan." I explained my plan to the patient and her husband. They reluctantly agreed to the scan.

Radiology took her to CT immediately. The husband said, "Honey, it will just show asthma and we can go home."

Her eyes widened, and she gasped for air. I turned up the oxygen.

The husband patted the patient's shoulder. "You'll be fine. We'll all be going home soon."

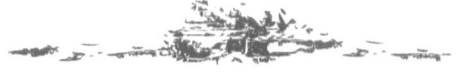

In the scanner, with a nurse at her side, the patient lay flat on her back. The scanner cycled, inching the beam through her chest after a bolus of intravenous dye. Radiology resident Duke Bradshaw watched the slices materialize on the screen. "Kelly, you're right. She has a large clot in her left lung and scattered clots in both."

As the scan finished, the nurse called to Duke and me excitedly through the glass partition. I rushed in. "She's looking worse."

"Let's get her back to ER and more help."

Duke helped us rush her back to the ER. He spoke with her husband. Under the bright lights, I took one look at her and saw real trouble. Blue lips in spite of high-flow oxygen, heart rate 120. "I can't breathe. I can't breathe. Do anything you need to do. I don't want to die. I'll do anything."

The husband leaned over to kiss her forehead. "How are you doing?"

She couldn't speak.

He shouted "Do something! You've done nothing to help her!"

I pushed the code button. "We need help. Get anesthesia stat and get that pulmonologist in here."

I grabbed the intubation tray.

Duke and I talked to the husband. We suggested he go to the waiting room with the baby. Duke explained, "Dr. McKay is inserting a special tube to help your wife breathe. She needs the tube and blood thinners to save her life."

"I'm not leaving. I don't trust any of you with her life." The baby screamed with him.

I said, "We don't have time to argue with you." I pointed. "If you must stay, please sit over on that chair out of the way so we can work on her." Duke showed him to the chair.

I asked a nurse, "Please get Pharmacy to run TPA down here to us stat. Load her with five thousand units of heparin and get the TPA going per protocol. We need to thrombolyse her before she dies." The nurse looked at me with questioning eyes.

"We need more nursing help in here." Staff responding to the code poured in. Annie showed up and took over. She always lowered my heart rate. I grabbed the laryngoscope and tube.

I talked slowly to the young mother, explaining the circumstances. "You need this tube inserted to help you breathe. There is a large clot in your lung blocking blood flow and causing your shortness of breath. The tube will carry oxygen support to help your breathing until the medicine can dissolve the blood clots. Sometimes the blood thinner causes severe bleeding, a risk, but this is the only treatment to help you. Do you understand?" She nodded. "You need this to save your life."

The patient nodded in agreement. The nurse made a note. I looked for her husband to talk to him about the risks and benefits.

He'd left the room.

"You'll feel funny from the sedative, like you're floating, then relaxation."

The patient's eyes filled with fear. "I can't breathe. Hurry." She struggled, hyperventilating and tiring. The nurse pushed drugs. First Versed to sedate her and create amnesia, then a paralytic. With bag and mask, the RT provided 100 percent oxygen until her muscles relaxed enough for me to insert the tube.

I made sure the suction was ready, the laryngoscope light was working, and tube was functional. "Ready. Cric pressure, please."

The anesthesia resident arrived in time to help. He pushed down on her neck, bringing her cords into view. Since I was already in the process of inserting the tube, I continued instead of turning the procedure over to him. I slid the tube in without difficulty. While I held the tube steady, he inflated the cuff and secured it in place.

Duke stood at my elbow. "Good job. Now that you have more help, Kelly, I'm heading back to Radiology."

"Thanks so much."

The anesthesiology resident took over oxygen management. "Slick tube placement, Kelly. What's wrong with this patient?"

"Pulmonary emboli. She deteriorated in CT, but not before we got the diagnosis."

He adjusted the oxygen and squeezed the bag inflating her lungs. "Her sat is eighty-eight percent. Is that better than it was?"

"Up a couple points."

I asked the nurse. "Is the TPA ready?"

She held up a bag of fluid labeled with the drug. "Dr. McKay, are you sure you want to give this? I've never given it for a PE patient, only for cardiacs."

"Yes, please give it. With a life-threatening lung embolus like she has, it's the treatment of choice. We often don't get the chance to intervene because most of them die."

I knew I should go talk to her husband but couldn't leave the room. "Get an ICU bed. Call the Medicine team since the pulmonologist wouldn't come in." Annie called while I listened to the patient's lungs and ordered another chest X-ray to check the endotracheal tube placement.

The nurse recycled the blood pressure machine. "Her blood pressure is worse, down to 80 systolic."

I fired off more orders. "Start dopamine at five mics. Double it in five minutes if her blood pressure isn't above 90. Bolus her with 300 mils of saline."

The anesthesia resident asked Annie to have a ventilator set up in ICU. "Let's move her up there right now before things get worse."

"I'm with you. We need the critical care team to take over." We had performed rapidly and appropriately in the crisis; now she needed ongoing care.

Annie hung up the phone. "They can't take her in ICU. They don't have a bed ready. They have to clean one for her, so we'll be doing ICU down here for about half an hour."

"This happens way too often," the anesthesia resident complained. "We're down here bagging people that should be on vents while they're washing beds. Hope they don't go to coffee before calling us back to say they're ready."

With the anesthesiologist at her bedside and some improvement, I left to update her husband. I found the tense man in the waiting room trying to give his baby a bottle of water. He seemed calmer. "Hospitals make me nervous. Junior here can tell. He's been screaming. How's my wife doing? I want to talk to her."

"We've sedated her and placed a tube in her airway to help her breathe."

The husband jumped to his feet, nearly dropping the baby. "I didn't authorize you to do that."

"I explained to you what we needed to do. When I looked for you to give you a report, you'd left. Before I placed the breathing tube, I explained the need and the procedure to your wife. She agreed to the care. Without it, she would have died."

"My wife was too sick to have understood all the consequences. She was in no condition to give informed consent. I'm a lawyer. Let me see her."

I took him to her bedside. He squeezed her hand. When she didn't respond, his expression changed from anger to fear. "Oh, my God. She's not moving. What's that running in her arm?"

"She is in shock. We're giving her a medicine to raise her blood pressure and a sedative so we can breathe for her and raise her oxygen level."

He shrieked, "This means she can't breastfeed. My son needs breast milk!"

"You'll have to feed him formula until she improves. We can help you with that."

"I can't take care of a baby. I have to work." He appeared in a panic, wild eyed. "I need to call her mother to come in and take care of him."

I handed him a phone.

He jerked it from my hand. "What have you done to her? I knew we shouldn't come to a training hospital where they practice on people." He stabbed the numbers and spewed a demand to his mother-in-law, then stomped back to the waiting room.

We eventually took his wife to ICU. He followed with an older woman gently cradling the sleeping baby.

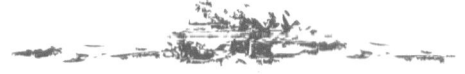

Mona arrived to work late and missed report. I didn't see her until late in the shift. She came out of Dr. Hunter's office with her face pale and her thin lips without lipstick to match the Red brand perfume that trailed down the hall behind her. She passed a med student and me talking with medics who had brought us a teenage diabetic in ketoacidosis. "With a blood sugar off the scale like that, he'll be a challenge.

The student asked, "Should we get two IVs started, one for volume and one for the insulin drip?"

"My thoughts, exactly." His quick, appropriate suggestions surprised me. I'd quiz him as we proceeded.

The patient's mother hovered at her son's bedside, answering my questions regarding his history. "Brian's been a real problem since his diagnosis a year ago. He was thirteen, not a very good student anyway, and the diagnosis decreased his self-esteem." The medical student listened and asked pointed questions. As we talked with Brian and his mother, the student and nurse started an IV in each arm and placed them on pumps. "He had a couple of insulin reactions and passed out at school, so his friends found out he was diabetic. He didn't want to pass out again, so he cut back on insulin." She handed me his sugar record. "This shows he has been running high sugars, 300–400. That's why he's here. I had trouble waking him this morning."

"Did he take diabetic classes?" the med student asked.

"We both did right after his diagnosis, but Brian rebelled. I found candy wrappers in his backpack, and he ate meals out with his friends all the time." She patted her son's hand. "He's lost weight and gets up often during the night to urinate. In the class, they said those were bad signs in a diabetic." Tears ran down her cheeks. "I told him if he didn't shape up, he'd go blind and be on dialysis like his dad."

"Did that help to get him back on track?"

Mother shook her head. "No. About four days ago, Brian got the flu and started vomiting. I don't think he's taken his insulin since then. He wants to do everything himself. I didn't know what to do and his dad is too sick to help us."

"Get the lab down here. I want an arterial blood gas and a stat capillary sugar when they do the draw." I turned back to the patient. "How are you, Brian?"

His deep, rapid breathing exhaled a strong acid odor. Brian barely responded, his face flushed. "I feel shitty. I want to die. Just leave me alone."

The medical student said, "Brian, I have diabetes. I'll teach you how to take care of yourself. You don't have to be sick like this."

Brian squinted. "You're shittin' me. A doctor who's diabetic?"

"I've been diabetic since high school."

Now I knew why my student understood proper diabetic treatment.

Brian said, "You fix me up, Doc. I'll do anything you say."

On the bedside test, Brian's blood glucose registered greater than 500. The lab called me with a critical value, a serum glucose of 940. The med student exclaimed, "Man, that's the highest sugar I've ever seen." After I calculated his insulin needs, the RN started an IV insulin drip.

I asked the student, "What are important aspects of this diabetic's treatment?"

"We've already started the insulin. I know he's dehydrated from the sugar in his urine carrying fluid with it, so he needs lots of intravenous saline." The med student's astute response surprised me. Other students weren't as attuned to appropriate care.

"What else?"

"We need to know his pH from the blood gas. He's in acidosis and, if dangerously low, will need bicarb replacement. Otherwise, insulin and fluid will reverse the acidosis."

"That's all true. Also, if we normalize his blood sugar too fast, cerebral edema and brain damage can occur."

"Really? I didn't know that."

"We have to bring his sugar down gradually. I'll write an order to check his sugar hourly and make adjustments in his insulin drip." After discussing care, the student and I re-entered the patient's room.

The student explained our treatment plan to Brian and his mother. Brian's lethargy interfered with his comprehension, but his mother said, "I'm glad this happened. Knowing you have diabetes and still became a doctor will give Brian more hope. Thanks so much."

The student wrote admission orders at the nursing desk. I read every letter to be sure they were correct before I cosigned. I complimented him on his skills. The young man smiled. "I love medicine. I'm glad to be here."

Mona approached us from down the hall. She stopped to glare at us sitting side by side and eyed the orders. "When you're done with the student, I've got a great patient for him, a crying three-year-old with a cut forehead."

The student looked up at her. "I'll be right there. Dr. McKay was just going over diabetic orders with me."

"In my opinion, we shouldn't be wasting so much time and medical resources on type I diabetics." Mona threw up her hands. "All they do is reproduce themselves and create more diabetics."

The med student's face paled. Nurses at the desk heard Mona's crass unprofessional statement.

Her statement shocked me. How could she say something like that? The statement was probably devastating to the medical student. I was glad the patient and his mother were out of earshot. I faced Mona. "Watch your tongue. That unprofessional remark warrants a report to Dr. Hunter."

"Don't you dare." She flipped a stray strand of her unkempt hair behind one ear. "That cut kid is in room 6. I'll meet you there."

The med student was still gasping at her remark. After Mona walked away, he said, "I didn't know people like her existed." The student became silent, obviously disturbed.

"Don't listen to that bitch. You're on your way to being a great doctor. Let me know if she gives you a bad time on your next patient."

After a couple of hours in ER, Brian had stabilized. His glucose level trended downward, and I turned his care over to the Medicine team. Later, when a code blue paged overhead to ICU, I hoped neither of my two ICU admits were coding. As ER physicians, we couldn't leave ER in response to codes elsewhere—we had enough to do. I found the med student free and sent him up to ICU to check on our patients.

He returned, his face ashen. "It was Brian. His sugar was 40 and he was seizing. They said something about the pumps being set wrong. I hope we didn't make a mistake on his orders."

"No. I checked them carefully. His sugar was 700 when he left ER. He was more alert and doing better. His IVs were on pumps, so it couldn't be a runaway insulin drip." I worried about his condition in addition to the impact a poor outcome in another of my patients would have on my probation. "That's awful. Was the Medicine team with him?"

He nodded. "And the neurosurgeon. They were examining him while a nurse pushed in a second amp of intravenous glucose to raise his sugar and stop the seizures."

A few minutes later, Mona found me in the dictation area. "Kelly, did you and that student ever screw up that diabetic kid. He's in up there FTD, fixin' to die because of you."

"It was nothing we did."

"You must have miscalculated his insulin drip. He looks bad."

"No." My words emphatic, "When he left the ER, his sugar was still high and falling slowly. Maybe the IV pump dispensing his insulin dosage malfunctioned."

Mona walked away shaking her head and rolling her eyes.

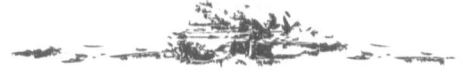

I welcomed the end of shift and waited with the off-going and on-coming teams assembling for Hunter's pyre. He asked me to present the first case. My detailed notes on the cases I thought he'd ask me to present to the group would guide me through his expected caustic remarks and interrogation. I stood ready for his onslaught.

"Dr. McKay, I strongly agree with your use of the thrombolytic TPA on this patient. You saved her life." I relaxed. "But, her husband is causing trouble for the nurses and interfering with her care." The husband had been such a problem, I'd expected complaints from him, but Hunter's favorable comments gave me a positive feeling.

Mona presented her septic ICU patient. Hunter grilled her on antibiotic use and how quickly the drugs were given. "Sepsis treatment *is* antibiotics. There was a significant delay in your orders. Next time, Dr. Maddox, I want antibiotics running in less than an hour after arrival."

Mona said nothing initially and then said, "Part of the delay responsibility lies with pharmacy. They were slow in filling my orders."

Hunter shook his head. "I can read. The fault is yours. Take responsibility and learn from my comments." Hunter turned to me. "Now, Dr. McKay, how about this young diabetic?"

I reviewed the patient's history and discussed our findings and treatment prior to transfer to ICU. I also complimented the med student for his expertise in front of the group.

Mona piped up, "If you both did such a great job, why did the patient code as soon as he got to the unit?"

Dr. Hunter's face turned to an immediate frown. "Dr. Maddox, is that true?"

"Yes. I was in ER with another admission when I heard the diabetic's sugar bottomed out. He's comatose after seizing."

Hunter's eyes stabbed me. "I have to review that case immediately. Critique is over. Get on with your day." Hunter strode out of the department.

I took the stairs up to ICU and found Hunter at the bedside talking to Neville Carrington. A ventilator cycled. Drips ran into both of Brian's arms. Hunter said to Carrington, "Do you think it's brain edema from being corrected too fast?"

"It's a little early to show much edema. Maybe it's just a hypoglycemic seizure and he is taking his time coming out of it. We're taking him down for a brain scan." Carrington appeared grim. "If there isn't a bleed and the contours are compressed, we will have to assume it's brain swelling."

When he realized I had joined them at the bedside, Hunter frowned. "Dr. McKay, this is not good."

I felt like I'd been struck in the chest and took a deep breath. "Let me show you the chart and my orders." I brought the record to him. "See, his last sugar in ER was still high at the time of transfer, and my order was for three units of insulin per hour. He had been stable with a slowly dropping sugar for two hours before I transferred him up here. His sugar couldn't change that much in such a short time."

Dr. Hunter scanned the sugars levels and handed the chart back to me. "Well, it did. You need sleep," he said, his tone accusatory. "I'll review the details and talk to you when you return to work this evening."

I walked away feeling defeated and confused by Hunter's critical intimation that Brian's deterioration was my fault.

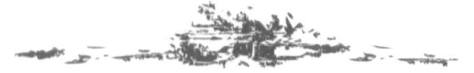

When I was back at work that evening, Hunter took me aside. "Your diabetic patient is alive, but not doing well. It's brain swelling from rapid correction of his sugar."

I gasped. "Dr. Hunter, I can't believe that. I followed protocol. Did you look at my notes, my orders?" I looked him in the eye. "I know I treated him right."

"Well, you were in charge. Somebody gave him the insulin too fast. I have set up a meeting with the ER attendings for tomorrow morning. I want you there. I also received a serious complaint from the husband of your pulmonary embolus patient that we'll talk about then. I hope you don't have any disasters tonight."

We never knew what would come through the door. I hoped for an easy shift. After about three hours of caring for too many patients, I dictated a stack of charts. Jen stopped by on her way home after admitting a stroke patient to the neurology service. "Kelly, you look busy. I'll just stay a minute."

Jen and I talked. Mona hung around and commented, "You're looking big as a house, Jen. It seems like I just heard you were pregnant and here you are popping out. Is it true that Kelly made the diagnosis? That's what one of the nurses told me."

"Actually, no. Even a neurologist knows when she's pregnant." Jen growled.

Mona went on her way.

I walked Jen to the door. "We need to talk privately. There are so many things going on here, I'm not sure what will happen next."

Chapter 29 Another Tribunal

Following morning report, I walked into the conference room near the ER at 8 a.m. Dr. Hunter and the other attendings from Surgery, Medicine, and Neurosurgery conversed as I entered. A lone wooden chair faced them. I imagined brush piled beneath the chair, burning. Flames from yet another ER pyre heated my face.

Hunter motioned for me to sit. In the preceding two and a half years, I'd heard of no resident ever being invited to such a gathering of department heads. Like an obedient dog, I sat.

They appeared as glum as I felt. An ominous feeling weighed on my body and brain, exhausted after running for the preceding twelve hours taking care of patients. As I looked from face to face, the image of a tribunal once again clarified my sense of being unjustly singled out and chastised for something I hadn't done.

Hunter started. "I asked Dr. McKay to meet with us this morning to discuss some serious patient care problems. Number one, you already know she had two elderly men in her care die for no apparent reason. In addition, in the past twenty-four hours, two more care concerns occurred. One young man may die. The other, a young mother, is not doing well and her husband may sue." Dr. Hunter folded his hands on the table. "Dr. McKay, please give us all a report on both patients. Start with the lung embolism case."

My gut clenched, but so did my fists. "First, I'm surprised and offended at being called before this group after providing excellent care and saving these patients' lives."

"Saved their lives? That's one of the questions here." Hunter's tone was brutal. "We need to determine if you are actually harming patients. Give us your side of the story."

I gave them a short description of the woman and the treatment with TPA. How I had called for consultation and the pulmonary attending refused to come in. "When I called a second time, he didn't even return my call." I discussed the literature on the CT pulmonary embolism evaluation and the use of thrombolytics and explained why I had used TPA.

"What about her husband?" Hunter asked.

"Her husband was a problem from the beginning. He refused to let me start treatment before obtaining the scan even though I told him she had a life-threatening problem."

Hunter tensed. "I spent an hour with him. He's a lawyer and is threatening a malpractice suit. He said you didn't give them a chance to choose treatment options, nor did you get a signed consent."

"I did talk to him. He wasn't listening. I talked to the patient. She agreed to the treatment, but she was so ill and hypoxic, I just got a verbal consent with a nurse witness." I stared at their all-knowing faces. "She was critical. I had to rapidly intubate her and give thrombolytics before she died. The husband was obstructing her care." I gave them an overview of my conversation with him after I had her stabilized. "I'll see him in court if he wants to play that game." I clenched a fist. "I saved her life in spite of his obstructionist behavior."

Dr. Biswell, the surgery chief, said, "Dr. McKay, that's not your decision to make. It's the duty of the attending physicians and University risk management to decide which cases to defend. Even if it isn't malpractice, sometimes we pay them off because it's cheaper than going to court."

"You mean to tell me I would have a malpractice case on my record forever because you wouldn't defend me?"

Hunter agreed. "Yes, sometimes that's the way it is. We call it the medical lottery. Some patients play that game and win big. We pay off a complaint because it's cheaper than a defense."

Carrington changed the topic. "Dr. Mc Kay, tell us about Brian."

"A teenage male diabetic entered the ER in ketoacidosis with a blood sugar over 900. I followed all the guidelines we're taught and slowly lowered his sugar, correcting his acidosis. After a couple of hours, he had improved and his sugar was coming down. His last sugar in the ER was still over seven hundred."

The Internal Medicine Department head glowered. "Why was his sugar only sixty shortly after we got him?"

"I don't have the answer to that. He was alert when nurses wheeled him out of ER, and his insulin was on a pump."

"Well, that's where we have a discrepancy Dr. McKay. According to ICU nursing records, the insulin pump was set about ten times higher than the level given in your medical student's admitting orders. Granted, ICU should have cross-checked the orders sooner instead of just documenting the setting, but how could you miss a factor of ten error?"

"I didn't. I think you're singling me out for no reason. Remember, I didn't set the pump. I wrote the order. I'm in my last few months of training. I have not changed the way I treat my patients. I am thorough and thoughtful. I assure you, I have done nothing wrong. It was set right. I checked it when I talked to him as he left ER."

Hunter stood. "This group has already discussed your patients from mortality and morbidity, and this makes two more. We don't know yet if they will survive. They certainly fit into morbidity with possible bad outcomes."

Dr. Biswell said, "Kelly, we all know about your problems and love life with Brett Warren. Maybe your personal situation is taking a toll on your professional competency. Maybe you should take some time off and get yourself back together."

That son of a bitch.

I stood up abruptly, knocking my chair against the wall. "I resent your condescending statement. I don't need time off. And I don't appreciate your sexist remarks." I looked at Hunter. "Dr. Hunter told me that one of you even suggested I might be on drugs. That's character assassination. I'll take a drug screen right now if you want. I do not use drugs. I did not harm those patients."

Hunter looked serious. "I have a question for you, Dr. McKay. Have you been treating patients without generating a medical record?"

I quickly answered, "No."

"I'm sorry you denied doing that. It's a lie. I recently found out you examined and treated a friend in the ER about the same time all these problems started. More bad judgment."

I couldn't believe they were exposing Jen's private medical record. Damn them.

"Not only that, I found you knowingly used a false patient name for some STD tests in the lab." Hunter's eyes were as cold as ice. "The tests were positive and not reported to the State Health Department. This will not be tolerated."

"Dr. Hunter, you are talking about a close friend of mine and just divulged very private medical information. This patient is a fellow physician with a sensitive problem, a problem that she did not want made public." I glared at him and spun to each face. "Now you all know. I certainly hope it won't be discussed outside this room. I'd forgotten about it. I examined her as a friend and as a professional courtesy." I gripped the back of my chair and leaned toward the table, furious at all of them. "Haven't you all done the same thing?"

"We aren't here to talk about anyone but you." Biswell again. "Your record was excellent until recently. It's hard to imagine that some of your behavior isn't related to your personal situation."

Dr. Hunter added, "Dr. McKay, it's my decision, and supported by the attendings, that you be placed on probation as of this morning. Furthermore, because the medical staff has lost faith in your ability to take care of patients, we are rescinding our decision to hire you into the chief position. I hope you understand. We can't have someone teaching medical students and residents who doesn't have the respect of the department heads. Dr. Maddox has a rough side that will need some work, but she was second on the list and has been given the chief position."

I clenched my teeth. Total shock swept through me and weakened my knees. I sat back down.

Be strong and calm.

"Dr. Hunter, all of you, I cannot believe you did this. There is no documentation of malpractice or incompetence on my part. Review of my records has been favorable."

"It's out of my hands," Hunter said. "We have to protect the ER, Harbor Medical Center, and the University reputations. Doing anything less would be an inadequate response to everyone's concern. Your probationary status will be announced today, as well as Dr. Maddox being named chief resident."

I looked at Hunter and each of the attendings in disbelief, all doctors I had worked with closely for years. I *had* respected them, but they were nothing more than a bunch of weak tag-alongs. "This is an unfair decision and you all know it. I will clear my name."

I threw my shoulders back, lifted my head, and walked out, my career incinerated by weak, morally destitute bastards.

Chapter 30 Fighting Back

At home, my fury erupted. I swept a stack of medical books off a table to the floor. I threw a cup into the sink. Shattered pieces scattered across the counter and onto the floor. How could those stupid sons of bitches think I did anything wrong?

They were worried about their own asses.

There had to be other reasons.

Hunter's issue was the ER residency program. I was a member of the first graduating class, and image and smooth sailing were everything in the competitive University environment. Success in the world of ER residencies was primary in attracting the best residents.

When I couldn't get to sleep, I sat looking out the window wondering what the future held. I finally fell asleep and then awakened in time to change clothes and head to the hospital before 7 p.m.

I waited for the critique to begin with my brain in overdrive, mulling over my disastrous situation. Dr. Hunter's eyes searched my face. I did my best to hide the pain and anger I felt.

Losing the job.

Placed on probation.

Patients dying. Lawsuit threatened.

Unbelievable.

Probation meant all my work would be questioned. It also meant all the personal sacrifice to do my very best had been trashed. Mona had gotten my chief job, and I might not be allowed to finish the ER residency after all these years of effort and stress. I wondered why Mona hadn't yet come over to pour alcohol in my wounds.

Lynn's hand pressed on my shoulder at the end of critique. She whispered, "Carrington called me today and told me what happened. Those sorry bastards."

My eyes teared. "Yes, I hate them. I dread seeing another patient while on probation, even one with a hangnail. I'm sure someone will find a fault with my care." We parted, but her caring left me with the strength to get through another shift.

I still had a stack of charts to dictate at the end of twelve hours and could hardly keep my eyes open. Dr. Hunter stood in the report area waiting for the residents and students to gather before starting his tirade. Not a patient man. He tapped his foot and checked his watch as I joined the group.

I presented the difficult cases in a systematic fashion. Easy diagnoses to validate. No one had died. Hunter's review was swift and clean. No bloodletting. At the completion, he dismissed the others and said, "Wait, Dr. Mc Kay, I need to talk to you."

I thought, shit, what good news will he give me now?

Hunter led met into a hallway for privacy.

My thoughts spun. Was it another patient issue? I hoped Brian hadn't died. I waited, anxious.

"Kelly, I want you to be very careful. Brett lost it when the Commission ordered him to rehab." Hunter appeared dismayed. "Biswell called me this afternoon and asked me to tell you to be careful. Brett didn't show up for rehab this morning. You may not be safe until he's locked up."

"Where is he?"

"We don't know. Biswell called Brett's lawyer, but he didn't return the call."

Anxiety and exhaustion left me transfixed, standing by Dr. Hunter.

In a few days, the life I had envisioned had vanished. Nothing left but a skeleton. No feelings. No future.

I thought of the empty exoskeletons of large beetles I saw each spring in Minnesota. After a metamorphosed creature took flight as an iridescent green dragonfly, the gray translucent shell it had emerged from stuck to trees along the lakeshore.

When the wind blew, the empty shells trembled.

Dead legs quaked but held firm, stuck in time.

Like me, stuck. Devoid of life. Devoid of a future.

I might as well be dead.

Maybe I should get in a plane and fly off like a dragonfly, forgetting my future in medicine.

After an arduous day and sleepless night, awake for too many hours after an endless night shift, now Hunter was telling me that Brett was angry and on the loose.

Be careful, Hunter said.

I cared little about my safety at this point. Come what may. I returned from despair and responded to Hunter's questioning look. "All of this is tough for me, but the worst is the probation. Brett and his threats are nothing compared to the importance of my career. I've driven myself to be the best for years, and now this. After I've had some sleep, I'd like to meet with you to see what I need to do."

"I'll meet with you any time to talk about probation requirements. Just call my secretary and she'll set up an appointment."

I went back to the dictation cubicle to finish my charts and left without a word to anyone. They could probably tell I was in no mood to talk. In fact, I couldn't even bear talking to Lynn.

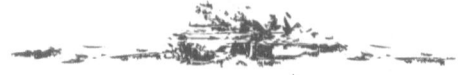

After awakening about 5 p.m., I felt a little better and tried to call Lynn before getting ready for work. She didn't answer. For three years, we'd communicated via voice messages. I left her a message to call me; if she didn't, I'd talk to her at work. The probation and losing the chief job were equally unbelievable in my mind. Maybe she could help me fight through the situation like she had during other crises.

I questioned all of my decisions at work and rechecked every drug dose. Work passed quickly with hours of chaos, crying children, cursing drunks, a waiting room ruckus, and violent drugged teens. I walked past three drunks on stretchers, already processed for detox, and stopped to say hello to Romeo, one of our frequent flyers. He'd been falling-down drunk but was good natured as usual.

"Waiting for a ride in the detox taxi, Romeo?"

His grin lit up the area. "Yeah, Doc. They're puttin' me on the wagon again and I just keep fallin' off."

The transport van that swept the city looking for drunks lying along the streets of Seattle had brought Romeo to Harbor before he became hypothermic or worse. I liked Romeo, and I hoped he would do all right at the detox center a few blocks away. I smiled and wished him well, but ugly thoughts swept through my brain. Now that I'd talked to Romeo, he might die because the mother of death had touched him. Typhoid Kelly; Kelly the Killer.

The first medical room had a full code in progress with more than enough people to help. I passed a stretcher carrying a comatose woman en route to ICU, an overdose, a suicide attempt. Inside the next room lay the lifeless body of a teenage male, an unrestrained driver ejected from a motor vehicle rollover accident. Resuscitation attempts failed. A baby cried from a curtained cubicle in the three-bed pediatric bay. I started my shift meeting an anxious, pacing teenage mother holding a crying baby.

My nurse reported the other two were toddlers with ear pain and fever but doing okay. I found the crying child wheezing and short of breath. She also had an ear infection. Her mother complained about waiting too long.

"When did your baby get sick?" I asked.

"She's always sick. Runny nose, coughin', has had a million ear infections. She's been bad about a week."

"Is there some reason you decided to bring her in tonight? Is she worse?"

"I couldn't get a ride till now." She gestured toward the waiting room. "A friend's waiting for us."

"Has she any history of asthma?" I listened to the little girl's wheezing lungs.

"Yeah, me, too." Mother coughed and cleared her throat.

"Do you smoke?" I already knew the answer. Her breath and clothing reeked of cigarette smoke.

"I can't quit. I've tried." She sniffled and coughed again.

The child clung to her mother's shoulder as I looked in her ears. "I need to let you know that if you smoke in the house and around your child, it's considered child abuse. It's essential for you to stop smoking around your little girl, and it's important for your own health to quit smoking."

The mother stiffened and glared at me.

"Her temperature is 102 degrees." I pointed to the nursing record. "She looks uncomfortable. When did you last give her Tylenol?"

"I need some samples. I don't have any money for Tylenol or her medicine."

I saw a pack of Marlboros in her open purse. "Tylenol costs a lot less than a pack of cigarettes. I'll order a dose of Tylenol to lower her fever and will start antibiotics for her ear infection. After an albuterol treatment, she'll breathe better." I wrote a few notes on the chart. "I want her rechecked in the pediatric clinic here in the morning." I marked the child's chart for a callback. "Be sure to bring her in before 11 a.m. We need to be sure her oxygen level is adequate. If she seems worse tonight, come back to ER right away."

"I don't have a way to get back unless a friend can bring us again. I love my baby."

"If you don't bring her to clinic, the Child Welfare Department will do a home visit and remove her from your care. Children with asthma can die without the proper care."

"You can't do that!" The woman hugged her child tight. "She's my baby."

"By smoking in her presence, you're jeopardizing her health. We'll help you take better care of her." I handed her the instructions. The thin little girl with curly dark hair breathed easier after a bronchodilator treatment and fell asleep in her mother's arms.

Annie saw me walking down the hall shaking my head. "What's going on, Kelly?"

"I'm so damn mad. I think any parent who smokes around an asthmatic child should lose custody. How can a parent buy cigarettes instead of medication for a suffering baby?"

"Kelly, you'll crack your jaw if you clench your teeth any harder. Try not to let things you can't change bother you so much. ER will wear you down before your years."

"It's too late. It always takes me a while to simmer down after a case like that."

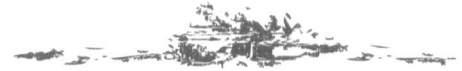

The triage nurse asked me to help her explain *triage* to an irate woman who had brought her mother into the ER in the middle of the night to be institutionalized. The family hadn't slept in weeks. They wanted Gramma "put in a home."

I watched a thin elderly woman scurry around the waiting room like an unruly two-year-old, picking through the magazine rack and sorting through items in the garbage can.

The nurse explained to the family, "If you're badly injured, Harbor is the place to go. You get immediate attention. But those who come for problems less life threatening, such as care of minor wounds, minor illness, drug refills, or a nursing home referral, have to wait their turn."

I supported the nurse's explanations. "Those with minor problems wait in line behind those who come in with chest pain, strokes, serious accidents, and gunshot wounds." We moved Gramma into a geriatric psych bed and settled the family down. A social worker obtained detailed information from relatives while I took a short break and found Lynn. She agreed to meet Sunday afternoon.

Jackson Hunter arrived for his review of the cases we'd cared for during the night shift. He tore into the group with his ruthless teaching skills, preparing us for the real world after training, a world I hoped I could enter the last day of June like the rest of the ER resident group.

I didn't go directly home. Instead, I drove to Shilshole Bay Marina. I had to verify whether Brett was in town, in jail, or at sea letting the wind carry his troubles away. Salt water dotted with sailboats sparkled in the morning sun beaming through scattered clouds. I drove along Dock C and recognized the *Chippie*'s mast from the roadway. Brett's car sat in the parking lot.

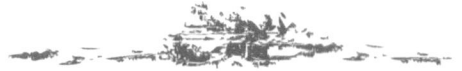

At home, I double-checked locks on the doors and windows, then turned on the television for morning news. I stepped into a hot shower to remove the night's sweat and germ warfare entrenched on my skin. From the bathroom, I heard the tail end of a news report. ". . . a young female dead of a stab wound to the chest. She'd been dead for a few days. A serial killer is still at large in the Broadway District. The area is a hangout for runaways." I quickly wrapped a towel around me and ran to the TV, but the report had ended.

I had hoped the Seattle Police Department would catch the killer before he acted again. Too late.

I called the SPD and asked for Detective Jones. He answered immediately, concern in his voice, "Kelly, are you all right? I heard about Brett and what happened at your apartment."

After a short conversation in which I convinced him I was safe, he told me the wounds on the bodies were similar. A stab into the second interspace between ribs two and three. A slice into the pulmonary artery with a sweep into adjacent vessels opened a bloody floodgate into the chest cavity. The victims quickly and silently bled to death.

"I just saw a television news report on another stabbing victim and wanted to talk to you about it. Where was she found? In Ravenna Park again?"

"No, closer to Broadway, just down the hill from the Deluxe Tap. When I heard your voice, I was afraid Brett was bothering you. Annie told me."

"I'm okay, but I'm worried because he didn't show up for rehab."

"You should be worried. Drugs change the way people think. He's probably desperate. Why did you call?"

"I know you can't tell me anything specific about your progress on active cases, but the two I treated had similar stab wounds. What did the ME say?"

"All of them are similar inside and out."

"It has to be someone who knows the human body, maybe an anatomy instructor, nurse, a mortician." I hesitated. "A surgeon. Could it be Brett?"

"Well, isn't that a novel thought." Cy said with surprise. "I hadn't considered him but will add him to the suspect list. Be sure to call me if he gives you any trouble."

Chapter 31 More Trouble

A few days passed. After an interlude for lunch followed by a walk with Lynn and Jen on Sunday, I switched to the day shift. Cy stopped by ER for coffee Monday afternoon. It was a day of the usual patient traffic with a couple of big accidents thrown in, too busy to drink much coffee.

For hours, the morning coffee pot sat on the warming element steaming the brew to a dark concentrate. Carrying two cups of coffee, Cy found me in the dictation room and sat in the chair next to mine. "After all my years of working long hours as a detective and drinking some of the most interesting coffee on earth, I couldn't drink what I found this morning. The stuff on the burner was too dark even for me. This is fresh. Made it myself," he said proudly with a little-boy smile.

I took the cup from him, unintentionally touching his hand. His eyes twinkled and the tiny smile remained. "I like it strong, like my women. None of that colored water without flavor." We talked while I plowed through some paperwork. He didn't stay long, but his visit gave me a boost, a little break from throngs of humanity in need. He brought no news on the stabbing death investigation. "I checked with the ME. Nothing new. Let me know if you come up with any ideas or if you see anything suspicious around the ER."

About 6 p.m., most of us were thinking about going home. We had gathered near the radio room, talking. A 911 call toned out, sending a Medic 1 unit to Marine Drive. "Unresponsive male. Possible suicide."

I didn't hear all of the report, but Annie was nearby. I kept my ear attuned to the radio whenever I was in the vicinity, anticipating what we might expect to be delivered to our door in the near future. "Annie, did they give an address on Marine?"

"Block C is what I heard. Sounds a little strange—why?"

"Could it have been *Dock C*?" My voice shook.

"Maybe." She looked at me with a strange expression. "Isn't that where Brett moors his sailboat?"

"Would he be that dumb?"

Annie retorted, "I don't know why not. He's screwed. He lost everything through his stupid behavior. He's a weak man. What makes you think he wouldn't try to take the easy way out?"

That poor bastard. I wondered if he had the courage to do it . . . to actually kill himself. Why didn't he ask for help?

My brain whirred yet seemed to be standing still. Not thinking about what I should be doing, what patient I should be seeing next, but instead remembering the good times Brett and I had had together. The fact that I had loved him. Inside, maybe still did. Not accepting what he had said to me and the horrible thought of disease he might have left with me. I hoped he wouldn't take me with him to the grave.

The Medic 1 doctor in the ER, assigned to receive all consults from medics in the field, beckoned me to come over. I stood beside him listening to his side of the conversation with the medics. He covered the receiver. "Kelly, the medics say it's Brett. He is down hard, agonal. They gave him Narcan and have him out on the deck now. They tried to tube him in the V-berth but had trouble getting it in, no room to work. It must be a circus. What a damn mess."

He kept listening to their cell phone report and periodically passed on information to me. "He's tubed now. IV's started. Loading into the rig."

Fifteen minutes after the initial call, a Medic 1 radio reported to the ER gathered staff around. "We're three minutes out with an adult male overdose. Initials BW. Unresponsive, intubated, pupils pinpoint. Given Narcan once with some improvement, repeating it now. Asking Medical Control for any additional orders."

Immediate response, "Continue current plan. We'll put him in room 3."

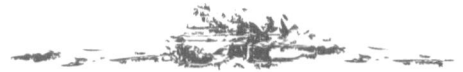

When I saw Brett, I felt a sudden wash of guilt. The feeling was short-lived, though. He looked like a bum with a couple of days' growth of beard, grimy. An arm dangled off the edge of the stretcher. Needle tracks along the veins, not failed attempts by the medics but instead his recent injection sites. Disgusting. Seeing him in this condition only reinforced my negative feelings toward him.

No tears.

I knew I shouldn't be involved with his care because of our past relationship. Before the ambulance arrived, the charge nurse assigned the ER Medicine resident to his case, who quickly spoke with the Medic 1 doctor. The two doctors worked over Brett. I manned the Medic 1 beeper while the other physician worked at the bedside.

People scurried around. Voices were raised. Orders were called out.

From the doorway, I heard the medic report, "A neighbor on one of the other boats found him unresponsive and called 911 from a cell phone. He was lying in the V-berth at the front of the boat, very difficult to reach him due to the narrow passages and crowded space in the boat."

The medic took a quick breath. "We found empty syringes beside him and an empty ampule of 10 milligrams of Lorazepam, the others unlabeled. Presumably narcotic, causing his constricted pupils. We brought the vials in with us for you to see."

Both Lorazepam and narcotics could cause sedation and respiratory arrest.

He'd tried to do it right.

I paged Jackson Hunter and told him what was going on. "I'm on my way. Maybe I can at least help with crowd control. I heard some of the radio transmission on my scanner."

Word spread. Everyone knew it was Brett and was unhappy it was one of us, one of the team. I heard a nurse say, "We should have helped him. We should have anticipated this. We failed him."

When someone committed suicide or tried to, those left behind always felt responsible, guilty. That's probably just what Brett wanted. Not taking responsibility for his actions right to the end.

Mona burst into the ER. "Where is he? Where is Brett?" She shoved me aside. "Get out of the way, you bitch. You did this to him." Mona plowed into his room, but Security held her back. She struggled to reach Brett's bedside.

The charge nurse whispered in my ear, "Want some distraction? There's a runaway teen here asking for you."

I looked at her quizzically.

"Name is Molly, a friend of that little street urchin you saw a few months ago that was drugged, beaten, and rapcd."

"Oh, that narrows it down." I couldn't stop my sarcastic remark. "They all seem to blur together."

"Kelly, you know, the one named Jamie. Remember the story about being picked up by the dude in the red sports car? Skinny little thing abused by her mother's boyfriend."

My heart skipped. "Yes. I remember her, well. She died in ICU, head injured and stabbed in the chest."

"This one asked for you personally, said she was a friend of Jamie's. She's here with some of the black-dressed punks. They are milling around in the waiting room but well behaved."

I entered the exam room to find a young female sitting on the end of an exam table, huddled in a thin patient gown, shivering. The gown draped like a shirt on a scarecrow. She looked up with a flicker of a smile in her clear blue eyes. "Dr. McKay, you don't know me, but Jamie said you're a good doctor. She said to ask for you if I ever needed to come here. She's dead now, you know."

"I know, and I'm so sorry. I hope they catch the murderer." I studied the thin girl's blank face below spiky black hair.

"Me, too. I need help. I can't pee it hurts so much down there." She pointed to her crotch. "A few days ago, I started getting pain. Now it hurts bad."

"Any other symptoms?"

"Itching. Burning, when it first started."

Molly grimaced as she moved. I listened to her heart and lungs, then helped her lie down on the table. I pulled her gown up. Her lower belly bulged. I listened for bowel tones and felt her abdomen. A full bladder, all the way to her navel . . . or was it a pregnant uterus? "When was the last time you passed urine?"

Molly put her feet in the stirrups for her pelvic exam. "Yesterday morning. I'm dying to go and I can't."

"Could you be pregnant?"

"No way. I got the Depo shot last month."

I sat on a stool near her feet and folded back the sheet, exposing her skinny legs and perineal area. One look gave me the diagnosis. Blisters and ulcerations covered her labia. Molly cried out when I touched her. Inside, more ulcers. Extensive lesions closed her urethra with swelling, blocking urination.

I rolled my stool to her side to talk. "Molly, you have genital herpes, a viral infection."

"I know who gave it to me." She slammed a fist on the mattress. "I'll make sure no one else gets it from him."

"You're contagious now, but even when the sores are all healed, you might pass on the disease to sex partners."

"Most of them deserve it."

"Herpes is usually worst the first time you get it. There is treatment, pills to keep it quiet." I waited for her response and asked the nurse to print an instruction sheet for her. "It often flares up with menstrual periods, stressful times, but sometimes for no reason at all."

"I really screwed up this time." Her eyes teared. "A girl I know has this and hers never goes away. What can I do?"

"I'll have a nurse put a soft little tube in to drain your bladder. It will hurt going in but will drain the urine and make you more comfortable. We'll have to leave the catheter in for a few days till the infection improves."

The nurse returned with instructions and opened a catheter kit.

I explained, "I took a viral culture and will treat you for all the common STDs."

"I'll do anything to feel better." She pulled the sheet to her neck with trembling fingers.

"In two days, go to the STD clinic here at Harbor on the second floor. The nurses will probably be able to remove the catheter then. You'll receive good care."

"I'd rather come back here to see you."

"My hours change a lot, and we aren't supposed to see medical follow-up patients in ER. Have them call me to discuss any problems."

I ordered a narcotic injection and a local anesthetic before her painful catheterization and wrote prescriptions for pain pills, antibiotics, and antiviral agents. She had no health insurance, no Medicaid coverage, and no money to buy the medicine. I had her talk with a social worker. The hospital pharmacy filled her expensive prescriptions.

About an hour later, I was rushing from room to room when I saw her shuffling down the hall. "Molly, you still look so uncomfortable."

"I hurt, Dr. Kelly, but not as much. I feel better. Thanks."

"Good. It will help if you can sit in a warm bath a few times a day. Be sure to take your medicine and follow up in the STD clinic."

She listened carefully. I walked slowly with her toward her friends. One girl asked, "Doc, did that overdosed guy they wheeled past us make it?" They others moved closer to hear my response. "He musta finally hit on some good stuff."

Chapter 32 Recovering

After work, I drove to Lynn's apartment instead of going home. We'd been too busy at work to talk. I touched the doorbell, and she snatched the door open so fast it startled me. "Kelly, how's Brett? I'm glad they didn't assign him to me. I just opened a beer. Do you want one while you tell me more?"

"I'm okay. Hunter told me Brett had started to wake up but was still on the vent when I left. Medics found empty narcotic and sedative bottles on the boat. And some other drugs they couldn't identify."

"Someone arrived just in time to save him. I hope, now, you can cut your emotional ties with him. It's a sad situation."

"I'll have that beer." I followed Lynn to the refrigerator. "When I heard the call to Marine Drive, a possible suicide, my heart flipped. I knew it was him."

Lynn popped open an icy beer and stuck it in my hand. "I don't suppose you heard the evening news."

I shook my head. "What, now?"

"Another body on a side street off Broadway. Stabbed once in the chest."

"Damn. Yesterday, Cy stopped by for coffee and told me a few more details on the autopsies."

"I think he's sweet on you, not just sharing death scene stuff. He never brings me coffee."

"I really like him, but I also enjoy the forensics. No leads, but the vaginal specimen DNA is identical on the cases. Cy didn't come right out and say it, but I think they have a couple suspects."

"You won't be studying for Boards tonight. Stay and relax. Try these." She handed me a bag of Kasugai wasabi roasted green peas. "I found them in an Asian market and love them."

The first handful of crunchy peas cleared my sinuses and gave me piercing head pain, like a surge of hot Chinese mustard. I drank a couple of swallows of beer and pressed the can to my forehead.

Lynn laughed. "I should have warned you. They're hot. Just eat a couple at a time and you'll like them."

I took another gulp of beer. "Now that I've recovered, I'll be more moderate."

"I'm addicted to them. Beware." We talked about my situation and again about Alaska. With everything piling on me at the hospital, I wondered if I'd finish the residency on time—or at all. Escaping to Alaska now sounded like the right choice.

On my drive home, my thoughts changed from personal issues to thinking about how the murders fit together. I wondered about the comment from Molly's friend. Did the druggies with her know Brett? Had he been prowling Broadway to buy drugs?

I fell asleep reading board review tutorials.

The next morning, Dr. Hunter gave the gathered residents and students a short report on Brett. He added, "No visitors are allowed. We're trying to protect his privacy. I'm telling you this as friends of his. Please don't divulge anything about him you observed. I think he'll be off the vent this morning."

Later in the day, Dr. Hunter found me in a dictation cubicle and sat down. "Kelly, how are you doing?"

"I think I'm okay." My flat tone matched my spirit.

"A shrink transferred Brett to the locked psychiatric unit on suicide watch. He agreed to go to the chemical dependency rehab program mandated by the Medical Licensure Commission. It's the only way he'll ever practice medicine again."

I said nothing, envisioning him standing on the deck of the *Chippie*, his wind-blown dark hair.

Next scene, near death in the V-berth where we used to make love. I sighed.

At least he wasn't dead.

Hunter's voice brought me back. "I'm personally monitoring all of your charts and dictations. With probation on your record, you'll have a challenge to finish the program with your classmates. There may be additional requirements to prove your competency."

"I haven't made the appointment yet to discuss everything you want me to do related to the probation. Things happened too fast yesterday."

"That's understandable. Like I said, just pick a time and call my secretary."

"Okay. Thanks for reviewing all the charts. If there's anything you identify as a problem, would you please tell me about it right away?"

"Sure, Kelly, the charts are part of the peer review process. All of yours will be critiqued over the next two months instead of randomly, as we have done on residents over the past nearly three years." Inside, those words didn't bother me; just more of the same. "The probationary period closes the end of May. That gives you one month to meet the imposed requirements before the end of residency June thirtieth."

Hearing such finality sent a shudder through me. The end of May could mean the end of the life I had planned.

Chapter 33 Another Blow

Every time I looked at the scar on my hand, I thought of my blood contamination combined with the risk of STDs from intercourse with Brett. I felt dirty, but a twisted sense of relief remained after the first set of follow-up blood tests came back negative.

Would they still be negative when I rechecked them in June?

The initial favorable report decreased my fear of disease, but the oppression of probation and loss of face in the medical community churned in my gut and seldom let up. Self-doubt weighed heavy. I lost my smile and more weight.

When Hunter and I met a week later, he reviewed a few chosen records with me. Although he had nothing negative to say, I no longer believed I had his support. His words were reassuring, but I wouldn't let him penetrate the shell I'd built around my emotions. Feelings of defeat surged, but I pushed them back. I trusted no one, including Hunter, the man I had admired.

I had to be strong to fight him and the other bastard attendings, but some days my reserve wavered. I felt weak and vulnerable after talking with him.

Carrington wandered into the ER one day like a lost soul. No one went out of their way to talk with him, especially women. Female nurses would just as soon castrate him as look at him. They'd heard his sexual innuendos too many times. He'd always seemed harmless to me. An excellent neurosurgeon with a shallow existence, looking for something, I wasn't sure what, except I knew he wanted Lynn. I thought he was really stuck on her and seemed to make up excuses to visit the ER even when he wasn't on call.

Nick brought a couple pounds of Starbucks into the lounge and made a fresh pot. I had signed out after a long day but stayed in the lounge to talk with him.

"I wish Lynn wasn't leaving town." He handed me a steaming cup of my favorite dark roast with cream, strong enough to help get me home. "After knowing her for three years, even though things didn't work out, I really don't want her to leave."

"She's taking a big step by going to Alaska, but that's Lynn. She wants to get as far away from her parents and Boston as she can."

"Going to Alaska accomplishes that." He sat back in his chair, looking pensive. "I'm thinking about having a going-away gathering for as many of you as can get there. I haven't used my cabin up on Sea Dog Island in the San Juans much since my divorce."

Hmm. I didn't know he'd been married.

"It's more remote than I'd like it to be. When I bought it, I thought it was perfect. No ferry service to the island, just water taxis and an airstrip."

I needed something to snap me out of my black thoughts and help me stop looking over my shoulder. Most of the nurses and other residents were friends. Mona was definitely not a friend, but I doubted anyone else watched my every move and questioned my medical decisions. Even though Neville was one of the tribunal, he was more of a friend.

"We need a party. That sounds like fun, Neville." A peaceful gathering on the water, away from the city, would be a perfect end-of-residency party. "What's with the name, Sea Dog? Some pirate?"

"No, it's named after one of my favorite creatures, sea otters. They're called sea dogs. We see a lot of them up there."

"When do you want to have the party?"

"The end of May. Before people start leaving town. I'll supply all the food, and everyone can bring what they want to drink."

"How much room is there?"

"Two bedrooms and a combined kitchen, dining room, and living room with a little fireplace. A screened-in porch looks out over the salt water. If everyone brings sleeping bags, there's room for a couple dozen if they're friendly."

"I need something to cheer me up. Just one big party! You'll have a lot of takers. I'll rent an airplane for the weekend and fly us up there with supplies."

He smiled. "That sounds better than a water taxi. Do you think Lynn will come?"

"I'm sure she'll be there. She doesn't leave for Alaska till mid-July."

"I haven't been up to the island since last summer. I need to clean the cabin. Could you fly the three of us early to check it out before everyone else arrives?"

"Sure. I'm always looking for someone to fly with me. I'll get out my maps and look at the runway layout and length."

"Kelly, it's a damn shame about you. You're a good doctor, better than the rest. I've seen this happen before. You've been railroaded." He sat down. "I'm trying to sort it all out. Hang in there. Don't let the vultures take you down. I'm on your side."

We talked a bit longer about hospital issues and politics before he walked slowly out of the ER.

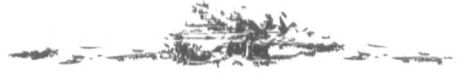

The next day at the end of report, Hunter spoke to Mona. "I want you to start July first. You need to get the new residents under your wing and started right. After a couple of weeks with them, you can take a few days off."

Mona beamed and brought her stout body to an erect position, almost standing at attention.

"I think you being here with the new group from day one is essential. I'll have a couple radios for you to wear and a cell phone for you to pick up the last week of June." Hunter fingered the radio, beeper and phone lining his belt

Alaska suddenly sounded terrific. It would have been difficult to jump right in and cheerfully instruct new residents with no vacation break.

I smiled.

Hunter's electronic umbilical cords would secure Mona to Harbor medical center day and night.

I might come out a winner in the end. I had lost the job through no fault of my own and would never forgive them. But now I hated this place more each day—and the two-faced pompous asses in charge.

I fled to my car. I had to get home since Lynn was supposed to meet me at eight for a burger.

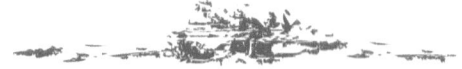

On the way into the apartment, I picked up my mail and threw it on the counter. I left the door unlocked for Lynn. She entered moments later. As I was slipping into jeans and a T-shirt, I heard an exclamation. "Kelly! Why didn't you open this?" She came into the bedroom carrying an envelope.

I looked at the return address. *Brett Warren, M.D.*

"I didn't see it. Frankly, I don't want to open it. See what it says."

Lynn ripped open the envelope and withdrew a sheet of white paper. A scrawl covered one page. She read aloud:

Dear Kelly, I'm detoxed. I've bottomed out, hate myself and everything I've done. They made me take antidepressants and after a couple of weeks, I think they might be helping. Anyway, I'm thinking of things other than myself now. They tell me it's a step in the right direction.

I don't expect to ever see you again, nor do I expect you to speak to me. I know I've hurt you beyond words and am truly sorry. I want you to know they tested me for hepatitis and HIV. I'm negative.

You are a wonderful person. Love, Brett

I stood like stone, unable to take a breath. "I feel sorry for him. It's very thoughtful for him to write, don't you think so?"

Lynn wadded the paper up and tossed it in the trash. "Kelly, rehab programs make them write letters of apology to anyone they've harmed. It's part of the spin-dry technique. All the druggies that go through rehab have to come to terms with their failings. That's one of the ways to do it. Don't be thinking about going back to him."

"I won't. I'm looking forward to Alaska."

I expected her to exclaim joy at my words. Instead, Lynn stood silent, grim faced.

"Kelly, I have bad news. The guys in Alaska called me, this afternoon. The medical staff secretary in Alaska read your application. Because you've been put on probation, they're asking you, off the record, to withdraw your application until the probation is rescinded. Until that time, they don't want you."

The Hunter and his bastard buddies had destroyed me.

Chapter 34 When Will the Trouble End?

Someday, I'd miss Harbor and the great staff, but right then I wanted the residency over, finished. The attitude among the senior residents was: *They can't hurt us now.* Unfortunately, that wasn't true for me. I had no assurance I'd meet the requirements, finish probation, or complete the residency.

At my last meeting with Hunter, he gave me mid-June for their decision. I couldn't complete the residency requirements on probation. At our weekly meeting today, Hunter informed me one of the orthopedists had submitted a written complaint about my care of a patient. He handed me a letter that read: *Dr. McKay missed a wrist fracture on a multiple trauma patient. It wasn't recognized until after he was out of surgery for other problems. He had to be taken back to the OR for wrist surgery that could have been done with the first anesthesia. Dr. McKay is a sloppy physician and hasn't reached the skill level a senior resident should have attained.*

Dr. Hunter waited for my response.

I flew into him in a defensive tirade. "It was an unstable patient in shock with a fractured pelvis that needed to be stabilized. I was more interested in saving his life than treating his swollen wrist."

Hunter's expression changed to anger and his eyes pierced mine in a magnetic glare. I couldn't look away.

"I agree it's my fault for not mentioning it in my dictation." I placed the letter on Hunter's desk. "But why didn't he take responsibility for missing it himself?"

"He's not under a microscope. You are. This is a new program, and every ER resident is scrutinized by other services."

"Do you have any other complaints against me?" I stiffened, hoping he'd say no.

"Yes, I do."

"What?" I couldn't believe I'd done or missed anything to warrant more complaints.

"I was sitting in a corner in the doctor's lounge reading a newspaper a couple of mornings ago. A table of doctors were discussing you. Either they didn't see me there behind the paper or didn't care. I sat and listened. They said you were distracted, not as sharp as you used to be, and are more argumentative."

"I speak up more than I used to. I must defend myself because of the probationary status. If I had not been put on probation and had it made public, I don't think this undercurrent of distrust would have occurred. I haven't changed anything in the way I take care of patients."

"Later, I talked informally with some of the group. We are meeting this afternoon. I'll let you know the outcome later today."

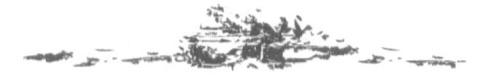

After critique I went to Hunter's office. He sat in his large chair and motioned me to sit. I perched on the edge of a chair in front of him, ready for my head to be severed, a sacrificial lamb. "Dr. McKay, I am sorry to inform you, I have extended your probation. You may not be finishing with your group, after all."

I felt like lunging for his throat but clenched my fists instead. "Do you have any specific complaints, charts for me to review?"

"No. They couldn't come up with any hard evidence but described negative interactions with you."

"How can I defend myself against nebulous complaints? How do I correct this?"

"Perform your duties to the best of your ability. I'll continue to review your charts, as will various department heads where you admit patients. I'll meet with you again next week."

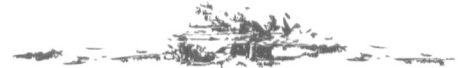

Depressed, but always the overachiever, I arrived at work early, stayed late helping others, and wrote detailed workups with elaborate differential diagnoses. I acted sweet to the damn attendings I'd grown to despise.

Hunter rated my next two evaluations acceptable. I tried to adjust to the concept of not having the teaching job I had treasured and being only *acceptable* after achieving honors in almost everything else I'd done in the past.

Lynn tried to cheer me when we crossed paths between patients. She talked about the party at Neville Carrington's cabin. "Let's leave for Sea Dog Island on Saturday afternoon, the day before the party. That way we can clean up and spend the night relaxing before the others arrive."

"I'm glad you're both willing to fly with me. It'll be a short, beautiful trip." I told her about the flight route and the uphill landing from the water. "I talked to Neville. He was anxious to have you come. He doesn't want you to leave Seattle."

"I know, but it's over between us. I'm leaving Seattle and him behind. Being on Sea Dog will be an escape too, something different for all of us." Lynn appeared tense. "I have some anxiety about spending so much time with him."

"I saw him putting a handful of invitations in resident mailboxes. I hope he didn't put one in Mona's or Brett's." I held mine up. "Leave it to him to come across crude. It says *BYOBABP*."

"What is that?"

"Bring your own bottle and bed partner." I smiled. "It's always something sexual."

"Will he ever learn?" Lynn shook her head in disgust.

"If he would just quit talking about sex all the time, he'd probably find a girlfriend."

"Maybe he'll strike gold in the next ER class."

Chapter 35 A Secret Revealed

Lack of enthusiasm among the residents nearing the end of the academic year prevailed. The thrill of making a new diagnosis or doing a special procedure dimmed with the ever-present anticipation of finality, counting days, counting hours, counting minutes till done. Packing up, moving, making travel plans, saying goodbye to people who were more than friends. People you had grown up with, cried with, suffered with. People you could discuss things with that you could never say to family.

Lynn's enthusiasm spilled over to those around her. She brought out the best in people. What a difference between working with her and Mona. At work, Lynn hung up the phone and exclaimed, "I'm excited. That was Howie. He and Shannon are coming to the party. That makes close to a dozen RSVPs. Neville invited all the ER residents, including Mona. He said he stuffed the mailboxes of nurses, surgeons, and medicine residents. I suppose he put one in Brett's mailbox, too. Not sure why since he's still in rehab."

"I'd hate to see Brett. I hope they keep him locked up till I leave town. I just wish my probation was over before the party and I knew I'd finish with the rest of you. Then, I could really celebrate."

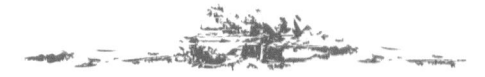

The Saturday before the party arrived. Neville and Lynn met me at Boeing Field at about 4:30. I wanted to reach the island in daylight. We had clear skies except for an onshore flow of wispy fog off the salt water.

Lynn and Neville placed all the baggage and party supplies on the tarmac near the plane so I could assess weight and load everything in balance for flight. I buckled two cases of beer and a case of soda on the back seat beside Lynn and placed the ice cooler in the baggage compartment with Neville's guitar case. I wedged in lightweight items such as our sleeping bags, small backpacks, hotdogs, buns, and chips anywhere they'd fit. Neville balanced the load by sitting in front with me.

We circled over the small island with a protected harbor lined with sailboats and motorboats of all sizes. In the distance to the northeast, Mount Baker loomed white and beautiful. The little airstrip stretched uphill from the water. After a calm, scenic flight, we landed before sundown on the narrow lighted strip.

Carrington's cabin sat west of the airstrip, about half a block from the shore, up a winding path. He had made a water-taxi trip a few days earlier, bringing heavy or bulky items, including box wine, beer, soda, canned beans, cheese, lunch meat, bread, bacon, eggs, and ham.

We lugged our load from the plane up the hill and nearly filled an old refrigerator that rattled and groaned but worked just fine. Winter inhabitants hung from webs in every corner of the cabin, some bigger than I cared to look in the eye. An adorable gray mouse scurried into the wood box by the fireplace. We shooed him out the door. The mouse or its relatives had left crumbs and pieces of wintertime nibbling scattered everywhere.

Neville opened all the windows to air out the place, then joined us on a walk to the beach. Low tide revealed interesting remnants of seaweed clinging to rocks along the shore. Seagulls fought over bits of broken crab and clams.

Later, we put Neville's brooms, cloths, Clorox, and a mop to use. We worked steadily for four hours and were too tired to gather wood for a bonfire on the beach, leaving that task to the group arriving the next day.

Neville lit a couple of candles, heated up some canned beans, and made sandwiches. We ate on the deck, looking at the water and enjoying the fresh air. He brought out his guitar and played classical guitar. Beautiful. Then he played folk music, singing in a wonderful baritone voice.

The evening breeze off the water brought the faint smell of fish, plus smoke from someone's campfire.

Inside, Neville built a fire in the fireplace, and we drank more. Neville played on and on, with our encouragement. He finally stopped for a rest. I refilled his glass with red box wine and noted how handsome he looked in the flickering firelight.

He sipped and stared into the fire. "Ladies, thanks for being my friends." Neville blinked. His eyes appeared moist. "I used to play guitar every day. It was one of my escapes, how I relaxed. I haven't played since my wife left me three years ago. Tonight is the first time. It feels good."

"Neville, you are awesome!" Lynn gave him a hug. "You should play all the time. It's a wonderful talent."

He continued as if he hadn't heard her. "I've been acting like a victim since Carol left. I didn't recognize we had a problem. I was happy and successful, teaching, cutting into people's brains, working very hard, keeping late work hours, bringing home lots of money. I thought she was happy till we were sitting in front of a roaring fire in our home in West Seattle one evening."

Neville touched his guitar resting on the floor beside his chair. "I was playing this guitar, singing a love song to her, when she put a hand on my arm and said, 'Stop, Neville. I need to talk to you.' I stopped. 'Neville,' she said, 'I'm leaving you. I'm leaving tonight. There's nothing you can do. I'm moving in with Megan. We're in love.'"

He stopped. Tears ran down his cheeks, glistening in the firelight.

Dead silence. We stared at him.

He went on, "'We're in love.' She repeated it. I couldn't believe it. 'Megan? You're in love with Megan? You're in love with a woman?'" He looked first at Lynn, then me, and threw up his hands. "Just like that, she walked out. Filed for divorce and asked for nothing. I haven't seen her since."

Carrington slumped back in his chair. "My heart went with her. I was impotent until I was with you last summer, Lynn. I say crazy things to sound positive about something that's been killing me. I've told no one this before. You'll have to forgive me for the way I've behaved." His shoulders shook as he cried.

Lynn was the first to move, the first to speak. She draped her arms around his wide shoulders and kissed away a tear. "Thanks for telling us. It's not your fault. You know it's not your fault." She moved around in front of him, held his face between her hands, then encircled his neck and held him against her body.

He hung his head, pulled away from her, and covered his face. She sat down beside him.

I squeezed his shoulder. "Thank you for trusting us." I took my sleeping bag, went out on the porch, and left them alone.

Chapter 36 A Funeral Pyre

The next day, on a beautiful clear morning two water taxis motored into the harbor. Seven people stepped onto the dock. The jovial crowd milled around, gathered their overnight gear, and hiked up the path toward Neville's cabin. The three of us left our vantage point on the waterfront and greeted them. Happy voices carried along the shoreline.

Annie came alone. Duke with Betsy, Jackson Hunter and his wife, Shannon and Howie, all traipsed to the cabin. I was surprised to see the Hunters and didn't feel friendly toward him since he'd failed to defend me to his peers.

Nerd surgeon Howie trudged along lugging his black leather doctor bag. Lynn called out, "Hey Howie, are you planning on making house calls for a little extra spending money?"

"You laugh, Lynn. Just wait. When you get shit-faced and fall in your drink, or step on broken glass, you'll have to beg me to do your stitches. I even brought anesthetic." Then he added, "But I won't use any on you."

Lynn relented. "With this group, you're smart to bring medical supplies. You may get to practice. Some of us still run with scissors."

Neville added, "I'm glad you brought it. I found my little metal box of Band-Aids rusted shut. I figured we could pour booze on open wounds to clean them and rip up sheets for bandages." Neville looked happier than I'd seen him in months. At the cabin, he offered drinks and snacks.

Late in the afternoon after wading in icy water, Duke and the others set up a volleyball net on the beach. A wild game without rules soon had participants lying on the cool sand laughing, being pummeled by opponents. Daylight faded. Stars sparkled above dark tidal water. Moonlight streaked waves washed ashore in foamy lines.

Everyone scavenged driftwood and dry logs. We produced an impressive pile of flammable debris for a bonfire. Wads of newspaper and small sticks at the bottom, then larger and larger pieces of driftwood, mixed with dry limbs from a thicket between Neville's cabin and the water. When we quit, the pile extended about six feet across and five feet high.

We laughingly called it our graduation pyre.

Dr. Hunter and Duke carried the large cooler down to the beach. They parked it upwind and a safe distance from the bonfire location. Others followed with party food, blankets, and chairs. Howie and Shannon disappeared into the brush to cut green sticks for roasting marshmallows and wieners. I ran up the dark trail to the cabin to use the bathroom. When the whoosh of flushed water quieted, I heard noises.

I opened the door and looked out to see who had followed me. I saw no one and went in the bedroom to grab a sweater. My backpack was open, with belongings strewn across the bed. Nothing appeared to be missing. I closed the pack and stashed it beneath the bed out of sight.

Who would do that?

From the deck above the group, I saw no one on the trail to the beach. I walked down and stood with the others, watching Neville splash fuel onto the pile. A noisy poof of volatile gases first ignited the paper and small sticks. Soon, the fire spread to larger pieces, sending sparks into the darkening sky.

Moonlight reflected across the water. A cold sea breeze carried smoke into a group sitting too close. A fishy smell in the sea air mixed with the bonfire smoke. We ran for clean air.

Delicious smells from our hot dogs and burned marshmallows blended in.

On a log near the crackling fire, Neville played oldies. Soon, happy voices sang along with him, stumbling over words and melodies.

Large logs carried ashore by fierce winter storms were lodged in the sand and provided perches. I sat on the end of one large log, away from the water and bonfire smoke, singing with Neville. I relaxed more than I should have with probation weighing on my mind.

I sensed movement in the darkness to my right. I strained my eyes to make out the figure.

Brett stood in the shadows, staring at me. My heart hammered.

When he realized I had noticed him, he stepped forward. Firelight flickered on his handsome face and dark hair. He looked striking in white cutoffs and a short-sleeved red shirt.

How long had he been there? Was he here to hurt me?

I felt exposed and vulnerable away from most of the group.

Brett walked over and sat beside me. Too close, his warm bare thigh touching mine. His arm circled my waist and drew me to him.

I stiffened and pulled away, not knowing if I should scream and run or listen to what he had to say. I looked into his face. Brett's presence overwhelmed me. His good looks. Our past love. His lies. His threats. Why had he come here tonight? What did he expect from me?

His eyes searched mine. He appeared worried, wounded, like a whipped puppy.

The music stopped. The others knew he should be in rehab and had threatened to kill me.

I moved away from him and stood to leave.

"Wait, Kelly, please." His eyes pleaded. He took my arm. "Wait. I need to talk to you."

I sat back down close enough to talk but out of his reach.

Neville walked over and welcomed Brett. "Look who came to join us."

Others exclaimed that it was great he could come. Someone tossed him a beer. Neville strummed, "Tequila." Drunks sang the favorite UW football stadium song louder than ever.

Brett joined in. He smiled at me, a gentle look.

My thoughts vacillated between fear, hate, his needle tracks, and the memory of our love. My heart raced in confusion and anxiety. Brett placed his unopened beer in the cooler and took a Coke.

"My rehab program ended a few days ago. I'll be monitored for drugs and alcohol for the next year, so I'm not drinking."

I didn't know how to respond.

I caught a glimpse of Lynn watching, frowning.

Singing, drinking, and toasts resumed. When Neville put his guitar down for a rest, Hunter asked Brett, "So what are you going to do now?"

Silence hung heavy as we all waited for his answer above the waves and crackling fire.

Sounding defensive, he said, "Right now, I'm just taking it day to day. I left Seattle yesterday and sailed most of the way up here. When the wind changed, I motored into the harbor at sunset. I'm glad I made it in time for the party."

After a couple more songs, Brett said, "Sorry I bothered you." He walked off into the darkness toward his boat.

Lynn sat beside me.

"I have to go talk to him."

Lynn shook her head. She grabbed my arm. "You're a fool. I thought you were afraid of him."

I ignored her comment. I took my diet Coke with me and walked rapidly down the beach, following Brett's disappearing figure. His long legs carried him swiftly away.

I hurried to catch up but lost sight of him when he detoured around a large driftwood tree half buried on the sand. Its skeletal limbs stuck up and blocked my route. In the darkness, I grabbed a limb and stepped on the big log to climb over. My foot slipped. I dropped my Coke and held tight to a gnarled mossy limb to keep from falling.

I looked back toward the dark water as my Coke gurgled into the sand.

Guitar music faint. Bonfire tiny in the distance.

I heard footsteps behind me. Startled, I turned around and saw nothing.

My heart pounded. I ran ahead. "Brett, wait. Let's talk."

A heavy hand on my back shoved me down against a large log. Someone twisted my T-shirt at the nape of my neck, choking me. I gasped and jerked away. I smelled Mona's perfume.

A searing pain stabbed into my right upper back.

I screamed.

The constriction around my throat tightened and blocked my air, my voice. I rolled and kicked. My heel connected.

My shirt ripped. I almost broke free, but I fell forward.

Another pain stabbed nearer my spine.

I screamed and wiped sand from my mouth. "Help! Help!"

"Kelly, you're done for. You selfish bitch."

I couldn't see her clearly in the darkness, but recognized Mona's voice and her perfume.

"You wanted my job, and now you're trying to take Brett away from me."

My chest hurt. I couldn't breathe.

Mona pushed me down in the sand and pressed a foot into my back. I tried to get up.

I heard running footsteps and got to my knees. "Help me. Brett, help me!"

Mona screamed. "I killed those bums to make you look incompetent and messed up that diabetic kid. You took my job. I wanted to show Brett and Hunter I was better than you. I'd loved Brett for years and after all I did for him, he went back to you!"

I rolled and grabbed her leg, trying to pull her down.

Mona broke free and kicked me in the side.

She seethed. "You bitch, Kelly. I saw him sitting in the firelight with his arm around you. I'm pregnant with his baby. I'll kill him, too."

She turned. Suddenly, Brett was grappling with her.

I scrambled to my feet, feeling weak and breathless.

Mona lunged at me from behind.

I twisted to defend myself. Her knee slammed into my belly. The force blasted a mouthful of saliva and blood into her face.

Mona spit in the dirt. "What have you done to me?" She wiped her face with her arm "You probably have AIDS!"

I lunged, grabbing her wrist with both hands, trying to avoid the long-handled scalpel she thrashed. She tried to bite my arm.

Brett held her from behind.

Mona twisted, pulling away. "Let go! You damn traitor."

Brett lost his grip.

"I protected you from those bitches who gave you drugs. They wanted your money and your body. I'm the one who loved you." Mona kicked at Brett and stabbed the air.

Mona broke loose and lunged toward me.

Brett grabbed her hair and jerked her backward.

With her in his control, I got a better hold on her hand and tried to free the scalpel.

Mona clung tight. She stabbed the air.

I twisted her wrist, turning the knife toward her throat. She fell backwards onto the sand. I collapsed against her, driving the knife into her neck.

Her voice croaked. Warm blood squirted from her neck, spraying my arms. She grabbed her neck, trying to stop the pulsing blood. Her words gurgled. "You thankless son of a bitch, Brett, I killed for you. I . . ." Mona broke away, gasping, and disappeared into the dark.

I kneeled on the sand. My chest hurt. I spit again and again. Blood dripped from my mouth. I couldn't breathe.

I tried to get up. My legs wouldn't hold me.

My vision dimmed. I felt sweaty and weak.

Brett tried to lift me. His hands slipped on Mona's blood that had sprayed me.

I coughed. "I think I killed Mona."

He gripped my shoulders. "She tried to kill you." He picked me up under the arms and dragged me toward the fire. "Help!" Brett stumbled through soft sand. "Help me!"

I heard footsteps running toward us. Voices. "What have you done to her, Warren?"

"Help me. She's been stabbed." Brett was out of breath but kept running, dragging me.

Someone grabbed my legs. They carried me along the beach and dropped me with a thud on the warm sand near the bonfire. I could feel the fire and hear steam hissing from moist logs.

I felt bubbling from my chest with each breath.

In the firelight, Brett looked frightening. Blood covered his hands and stained his white shorts. He appeared stunned, scared.

Duke pulled him away from me and struck him in the face.

Brett fell to his knees. He tried to get up. Others stepped forward. Blows rained down on him. Brett raised both arms to deflect the blows. He gasped, "I didn't do it. Help her. She's been stabbed. It's bad."

I coughed and gurgled. "I can't breathe." Logs crackled near me. Sparks drifted into a black sky and meshed with stars. Smoke choked my breath.

"I didn't do it. Kelly, tell them I didn't do it. Mona went psycho and stabbed her."

I nodded. My chest gurgled with each breath. Duke yelled to the group, "Mona went crazy. She stabbed Kelly. Give us some help."

Coughing, spewing blood, I sat up. "I can't breathe." I searched the faces of my friends. "Help me. I think I'm dying. Mona said she killed my patients."

Howie lifted my shirt. "Shit. She has two chest wounds. Get her up to the house. I have IVs in my bag."

Hunter kneeled beside me. His fingers pressed on my carotid artery, fingered my trachea, looked at my wounds. "IVs?" Hunter's voice boomed. "Goddammit, what she needs is blood and the helicopter." He punched a cell phone. "This is Hunter. Dispatch the Life Flight helicopter to Sea Dog Island airstrip stat! Bring a 32-chest tube with a water seal and six units of O negative blood. Dr. McKay's been stabbed. Hurry. She's critical. We'll be on the runway with her."

Lynn ordered, "Clear the way. Get her to the cabin."

Brett and others hoisted me. Hands gripped my legs and torso, lifting and jostling me with each running step up the winding path. They laid me on the kitchen floor. Heat from the noisy refrigerator motor felt good against my skin. The linoleum was cold, icy cold on my legs.

I shook uncontrollably.

Lying flat on my back, I looked up into a ring of worried faces. "What happened, Kelly?" someone asked. "Can you talk?"

I held my chest and tried to breathe. "Mona stabbed me with a scalpel." I took a breath. "She killed the young women to protect Brett." When I coughed, more blood spewed out. "He was hitting on them for sex and drugs. She was jealous." I felt faint, losing consciousness. I fought the feeling. Took a deep breath.

Brett said, "Mona confessed. She killed some old guys in the ER, too, and said something about a diabetic kid. She wanted to make Kelly look bad."

Hunter blew up. "Where is Mona? Where's that goddamn psychopath?"

Lynn's frightened eyes looked down at me. She wiped blood off my face and away from my mouth with a cool cloth. "Hang on, honey. Hang on. Don't die. Please don't die. Breathe. Howie's getting things ready." She squeezed my arm.

Brett's blurry face appeared close to mine. He looked directly into my eyes. "Kelly, we're going to help you." I felt his hand on my neck and jerked away. "I won't hurt you, Kelly."

With a stethoscope in his ears, Howie ripped my shirt up the front. "No breath sounds on the right. Her trachea's deviated. She has a tension pneumo. Hurry! We have to needle her chest."

Even in shock and struggling to breathe, I hated having my chest and burn scars exposed.

Howie rummaged in his bag. "Here's a fourteen-gauge Heimlich valve." He handed it to Brett. "Needle her, now, or I'll do it."

I looked into blurry faces.

Brett's cold fingers counted ribs and chose the proper site. I tried to scream but could only gasp when he shoved the nail-sized needle between two ribs into my upper chest. Air gushed out.

Suddenly, I could breathe better.

Howie leaned in. "Help me turn her over. Let me see her back."

I tried to turn but couldn't. Hands helped me. I heard Howie's voice. "One wound near the right scapula and another below it. Shannon, Annie, tape occlusive dressings over the stab wounds. Kelly, take a deep breath!"

I tried to breathe deep. It hurt. I coughed. "Help me. Don't let me die. I'm so cold."

They turned me to my back again.

"Throw some sleeping bags over her." Howie said, "Get two IVs going. Damn, I only brought two liters of saline. That's not enough."

Needles poked both arms. The sharp jabs felt good. I was still alive.

Brett whispered in my ear. "I'm sorry, Kelly. So sorry." A tear dripped onto my face. He kissed my cheek and warm fingers squeezed my hand.

Cold. Shaking. Cold. Where am I? Can't breathe. Can't breathe.

Voices far away . . . far away . . .

Brett's voice. "She's fading. Squeeze the fluid bags."

Pain, sharp chest pain.

Jackson Hunter's voice. I opened my eyes to Hunter's worried face close to mine. "Kelly, your lung collapsed. Brett put in a Heimlich valve." I closed my eyes. Too tired. Fading. "The flight team is coming. Fight, girl. Hang in there. Fight. We're moving you down to the airstrip."

Don't care.

I'm dying. I can't breathe.

Smoke. I'm at the bonfire, floating into the pyre, my funeral pyre. I feel hot, so hot.

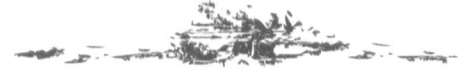

Whup-whup-whup. Bright lights.

Coughing. Can't breathe.

A flight nurse said, "Kelly, we're going to put a tube down. We have to keep your airway open. Your oxygen is too low. I'm giving you drugs."

Arm burns.
Drifting. Floating.
Darkness.

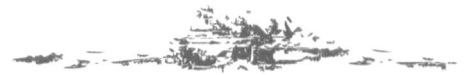

A soft repetitive whooshing entered my senses. My chest and throat hurt. I opened my eyes. Where am I? What happened? When I tried to talk, nothing came out.

I couldn't move. Hands tied.

Panic.

Help me! Let me go. I tried to scream. Nothing came out.

My eyes didn't focus, and then I saw Brett's face.

I jerked away. Kicked.

Couldn't get away. So afraid.

Brett squeezed my hand. "Kelly, it's okay. You're going to be all right."

A blurry nurse loomed into view. "You're on a ventilator, Kelly. Don't fight it. When you're more awake, we can pull out the tube." I felt something hot surge into my arm vein.

My chest quit hurting. I couldn't move.

Sleep.

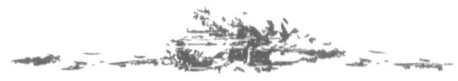

Voices. My mother crying. My mother? I looked around. My mother and my sister Kris stood beside me, Dr. Hunter with them. "Hey, Kelly. Wake up. Your family just arrived." His voice sounded cheery. Hunter drew my mother closer to the bed. Kris took my hand. "Kelly, Mom and I came to be with you. We're here."

Mom's arms were around me. "I love you, honey. Please don't die like Daddy. We need you. I'm so proud of you."

My body convulsed with sobs. Mom actually came to be with me.

"Now, don't you start crying or the whole bunch of us will be." Kris squeezed my hand. "Dr. Hunter says you're doing fine. Just rest and get well."

My eyes opened wide. I fought to get loose.

Fear. Mona. What if she comes in here and I'm connected to all these tubes? I can't get away.

"It's all right, baby." Mom gently hugged me, trying to avoid the monitor wires and tubes everywhere. "We won't let anyone hurt you."

Then, I remembered.

I killed Mona.

I looked at Dr. Hunter and pointed at the tube. I bent forward toward my tied hand and tried to grasp the tube protruding from my mouth. I mouthed the words. "Out. Out."

"I'll see what your surgeon says. I think she'll remove it soon. You've had six units of blood. The chest X-ray is looking better. You didn't need a thoracotomy, but you still have a tube in the right side."

I struggled to get loose.

"You're still at risk for collapsing that lung," Hunter explained. "We will get the ET tube out soon, but the chest tube will be in for about a week."

A nurse came with a syringe and pushed something into my intravenous line.

Floating away.

Nightmares. Dad's face. Fog in the cockpit. Fire.

EPILOGUE

On Sea Dog Island at sunrise the following day, local residents and police found Mona's body. My attack on her was judged self-defense.

During the next month, I spent most of the time being babied, taking walks, and getting to know Mother and Kris again after so much time apart during my schooling. A more positive relationship with my mother evolved after she experienced my brush with death this time. I gradually felt strong enough to enjoy excursions with them to Seattle-area highlights.

Cy Jones came to visit. Mona's confession allowed him to close many unsolved cases, with possibly more to be determined.

My final image of Brett's blurry face at my bedside in the ICU was from a time when I couldn't scream and couldn't run. My anxiety attacks accelerated after the injuries, related to being tied down and trapped on that damn ventilator, unable to escape. Without sedation, I would have ripped out the tube and run.

I called Brett after a couple of weeks at home in my apartment and thanked him for saving my life. Our awkward, short conversation helped provide closure for me. I didn't want to see him but knew I'd never forget his touch. He, too, had been caught in the black web of a psychopath.

I got my FAA medical clearance to fly again. Other than a few small scars on my chest and an occasional anxiety attack, I felt more rested than I'd been in years. My last set of blood tests confirmed no HIV nor hepatitis.

The chairman of the Mortality and Morbidity Committee sent me flowers.

Bastards.

The attending review committee members sent a sincere apology for putting me on probation.

Spineless bastards.

When I had an outpatient medical evaluation with a new surgical trauma attending, she assured me I would need at least another month to recover before returning to work. I warned her about the sexist old boys' club and wished her well in her new position. She looked like someone who could handle herself in any setting—six feet tall, with long blonde hair and long legs that I knew Neville Carrington would be admiring.

After the appointment with her, I met with Dr. Hunter in his office. I rested in the same chair where I'd once sat, dismayed, when he said I could lose the chief resident position and might not complete the program. Now I didn't want the damn job.

Dr. Hunter leaned across his desk and handed me an envelope containing the residency diploma. He sighed and folded his hands on a stack of medical journals. "Kelly, I'll never forgive myself for not defending you. Please accept my apology. You are the best resident and the best selection for the teaching position. I would love to work with you for another year and try to make up for the disastrous treatment you received here. Will you accept the position after taking a couple months off?"

I turned him down cold.

I wanted to leave Seattle and the chaos behind.

Someday, I'd return to play in the beautiful city I hadn't been able to fully appreciate because of my long work hours. My sister offered to store my car and a few personal items. I gave my second-hand furniture to an intern, like a resident had done for me three years earlier.

Lynn moved to Alaska and called me daily. The twenty-four hours of daylight captivated her. She loved it. The hospital in Anchorage offered me an ER job, starting whenever I felt ready.

Kris and Mom dropped me at the entrance to the Alaska Ferry Terminal. Kris told me her wedding was off and she'd keep me posted when they worked things out. I hoped she'd be happy and learn to choose better men than I had.

I waved goodbye. The country girls from Minnesota drove off in my Subaru and disappeared in traffic.

Shortness of breath slowed my walk up the ramp onto the ferry. It reminded me of my ordeal and blood loss. I rested at the railing and watched. Strong pulsing engines churned to life, moving the large vessel away from the dock.

Like the ferry, I was free.

Free.

Free from the bondage of intense hours in ER.

Free from Mona. Free from Brett. Free from hepatitis and AIDS.

The sun dropped low on the horizon and turned wisps of evening fog to orange. The ferry picked up speed in fresh air untainted by exhaust. Seagulls screeched and wheeled overhead. Some dived to the foamy wake, where they fought over a flotilla of edible scraps thrown by passengers.

Northward bound.

The peak of Mount Baker turned to pink ice cream in the fading sun. The Cascade Mountains disappeared from view. A friendly honk from a motorboat brought me back from faraway thoughts. The boat sped past. A young woman with wind-blown hair and an amazing tan line mooned us.

Men cheered and waved from the ferry.

The two couples on the powerboat boogied and honked a few more times. They disappeared, trailing a large skull and crossbones flag high off their stern.

I was wearing my going-away present from Hunter, an orange baseball cap stitched with *Fly Alaska*.

That's exactly what I planned to do.

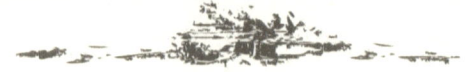

THE END

Questions and Topics for Discussion

1. Did the plot of *Deadly Pyre* keep you interested?

2. Were the emergency room scenes realistic and understandable? Did they give you a feeling of being there?

3. Major themes in the book are workplace sex discrimination, false accusations and deception. How do you think her focus on saving lives helps Kelly deal with stress? How would you deal with similar circumstances?

4. How does Kelly survive the exhaustion and injustice in her medical training?

5. Did you enjoy the flying scenes? Did you follow the action? Would you like to become a pilot?

6. Did the book end the way you expected?

7. What did you like best about *Deadly Pyre*?

8. Are you interested reading the next book, *Deadly Spin*, set in Alaska?

Afterword

Thank you for reading *DEADLY PYRE*. I hope you enjoyed it. If you did:

- Help others find this book. Tell your friends.
- Write a review at your favorite retailer.
- Like my Facebook page: http://www.facebook.com/betty.kuffel
- Visit my website: http://bettykuffel.com

I enjoy discussing my novels with book club readers. If your group is interested in talking with me during your discussion of *DEADLY PYRE*, please contact me at

MontanaSunriseBooks@gmail.com

Betty Kuffel

ACKNOWLEDGEMENTS

Many thanks to Dennis Foley and friends in Authors of the Flathead who have been instrumental in guiding my efforts. Debbie Burke was key in bringing this book through many iterations to completion. Special thanks to her and my other critique members who remain generous with their time and skills: Deborah Epperson, Marie Martin, Phyllis Quatman, Susan Purvis and Ann Coleman.

I also thank my husband Tom for his support and publication formatting. Editor Kathy McKay provided important advice.

About The Author

Betty Kuffel:
Dr. Kuffel is a pilot and retired ER physician who lives in Montana. Medical and wilderness experiences, flying, dog sled racing in Alaska, and surviving a plane crash in the mountains of Idaho fuel her writing.

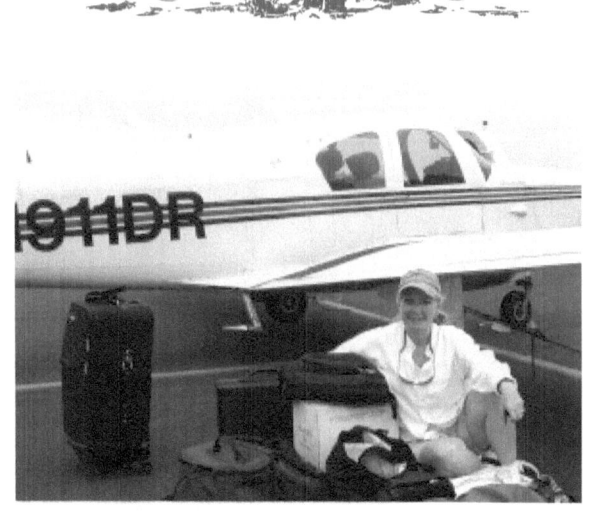

Excerpt DEADLY SPIN – Book 2 – Alaska

Chapter 1 Birdman

Crisscrossed restraints pinned a writhing young man face down on a stretcher. Medics and two police officers guided their patient toward waiting night staff in Anchorage Regional ER. A disheveled medic asked, "Where do you want him, Doc?"

"In lockdown." I pointed down a long hallway.

Vic's muscles strained his blue scrubs as the tall ex-military RN gripped the stretcher to help the medics roll it along. "I knew who it was when I heard your radio report. We haven't seen him for a while."

As ER doc for the night, I followed my next patient to a room where leather-cuffed straps dangled from a bed bolted to the floor. Grimy hands cuffed behind his back grabbed blindly at his captors. He spewed profanity and whipped his long hair from side to side as the entourage entered the room.

One of the police officers assisting the medics said, "This looks like a secure spot where he can't hurt anyone."

Vic eyed the unruly patient. "Yeah, except us."

I walked closer for a better look "I thought work in Alaska would be peaceful."

Vic told the group, "This is Dr. McKay's first week here on the job. She came from a big trauma center in Seattle to relax."

"We wouldn't want you to get bored." An officer patted the patient's leg. "Tonight, this here nice man was making a disturbance at the Great Alaskan Bush Company, a topless joint downtown."

"The officers called us for backup." A medic at the patient's head spoke calmly. "You'll find a few bruises on Birdman. It took all of us to get him under control. He was screaming about the naked women shaking their boobies."

"I'll remove his cuffs when you're ready." An officer held up a key. "I've known him for years. He can be very nice, but this time he gets the wingnut of the week award."

Vic's six-three frame shielded me from the patient. "Let's calm him down before you get too close, Doc. Last time, he nearly broke a nurse's neck when he grabbed her hair." Vic directed the team, "We need to strip him and flip him onto the bed. We'll all be safer after he's locked in five-point leathers. I'm thinking we need two more guys to help us so nobody gets hurt."

The patient wailed. "Don't tie me down. Let me go and I'll get the hell out of here."

I said over the intercom, "We need two strong men to help us move a patient."

A voiced answered. "Security and Rob will be there in a minute."

Vic orchestrated the move. I'd helped manage violent patients many times during my training at Harbor Medical Center in Seattle, but I stood back and admired the former Marine in action. One look at Vic and most rowdy patients would do whatever he asked, but not this guy.

"Let's remove his jeans while he's still face down. Untie one leg at a time. Once he's undressed, wrap the leather cuffs around each ankle." Vic motioned to an officer. "I'll let you know when I'm ready to have you unlock his handcuffs. After that, you secure the waist belt, loop the cuffs, and attach each side to the bed frame.

While I waited out of reach, my anxiety rose just watching them.

"Dr. McKay, would you remove the spider straps when we have him under control?"

I nodded and moved closer.

Vic positioned himself at the patient's head. "I'll take the upper body. Rob, you take one arm, Security the other, a medic on each leg. On the count of three, we'll turn him over onto the bed and lock him to the frame."

Vic spoke in a calm voice. "John, you can make this easy on everyone, including yourself, by cooperating."

The patient screamed, "Go to hell!"

"If that's the way you feel, okay." Vic asked his cohorts, "Are you ready?"

In a valiant fight, John wrenched his torso free from Vic's grasp and kicked a medic. The patient's agitation and profanity spiked when his legs and body were fully restrained. Staff members vice-gripped his arms while Vic set about removing the man's turtleneck. He gave up when the patient clamped his chin down and then tried to bite him.

I hadn't expected such violence on my first night at work after moving to Alaska. I'd finished ER training three months earlier and recovered from near-fatal stab wounds. I say "recovered," but the sight of this violence clenched my gut and triggered anxiety I'd tried to suppress. Hiking and flying around the wilderness 31area had strengthened me and lowered my stress, but I wasn't quite ready for this.

Tonight, I had the urge to run.